W9-AFY-113

MRI at a Glance

Catherine Westbrook MSc PgC(HE) FHEA DCR(R) CTCert

Senior Lecturer and Post-graduate Pathway Leader
Faculty of Health and Social Care
Anglia Ruskin University
Cambridge, UK

Second Edition

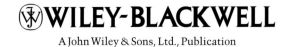
WILEY-BLACKWELL

A John Wiley & Sons, Ltd., Publication

This edition first published 2010
© 2010 Catherine Westbrook and 2002 Blackwell Science Ltd

Blackwell Publishing was acquired by John Wiley & Sons in February 2007. Blackwell's publishing programme has been merged with Wiley's global Scientific, Technical, and Medical business to form Wiley-Blackwell.

Registered office
John Wiley & Sons Ltd, The Atrium, Southern Gate, Chichester, West Sussex,
PO19 8SQ, United Kingdom

Editorial office
350 Main Street, Malden, MA 02148-5020, USA

For details of our global editorial offices, for customer services and for information about how to apply for permission to reuse the copyright material in this book please see our website at www.wiley.com/wiley-blackwell.

The right of the author to be identified as the author of this work has been asserted in accordance with the Copyright, Designs and Patents Act 1988.

All rights reserved. No part of this publication may be reproduced, stored in a retrieval system, or transmitted, in any form or by any means, electronic, mechanical, photocopying, recording or otherwise, except as permitted by the UK Copyright, Designs and Patents Act 1988, without the prior permission of the publisher.

Wiley also publishes its books in a variety of electronic formats. Some content that appears in print may not be available in electronic books.

Designations used by companies to distinguish their products are often claimed as trademarks. All brand names and product names used in this book are trade names, service marks, trademarks or registered trademarks of their respective owners. The publisher is not associated with any product or vendor mentioned in this book. This publication is designed to provide accurate and authoritative information in regard to the subject matter covered. It is sold on the understanding that the publisher is not engaged in rendering professional services. If professional advice or other expert assistance is required, the services of a competent professional should be sought.

Library of Congress Cataloging-in-Publication Data
Westbrook, Catherine.
 MRI at a glance / Catherine Westbrook. – 2nd ed.
 p. ; cm. – (At a glance series)
 Includes index.
 ISBN 978-1-4051-9255-2 (pbk. : alk. paper)
 1. Magnetic resonance imaging – Outlines, syllabi, etc. 2. Medical physics – Outlines, syllabi, etc.
I. Title. II. Series: At a glance series (Oxford, England)
 [DNLM: 1. Magnetic Resonance Imaging. WN 185 W523m 2010]
 RC78.7.N83W4795 2010
 616.07′548–dc22   2009016225

A catalogue record for this book is available from the British Library.

Set in 9/11.5pt Times by Graphicraft Limited, Hong Kong
Printed in Singapore

1 2010

Contents

Preface

MRI at Glance is one of a series of books that presents complex information in an easily accessible format. This series has become famous for its concise text and clear diagrams. Since the first edition of *MRI at a Glance* was published, the series has been updated to include colour diagrams and a new layout with text on one page and diagrams relating to the text on the opposite page. In this way all the information on a particular topic is summarized so that the reader has the essential points at their fingertips.

The second edition has been updated to reflect the new layout of the series as a whole. Colour diagrams are now included and I have updated the text to incorporate more detail on topics such as K space (which now includes the famous Chest of Drawers analogy) and other developments like parallel imaging, EPI and diffusion. Each topic is presented on two pages for easy reference and large subjects have been broken down into smaller sections. I have included simple explanations, analogies, bulleted lists, tables and plenty of images to aid the understanding of each topic. There are also appendices on acronyms, abbreviations and artefacts. The glossary has also been significantly expanded.

This book is intended to provide a concise overview of essential facts for revision purposes and for those very new to MRI. For more detailed explanations the reader is directed to *MRI in Practice* and *Handbook of MRI Technique*. Indeed the diagrams and images in this book are taken from these other texts and *MRI at a Glance* is intended to compliment them.

I hope that everyone enjoys the new format. Happy Learning!

Acknowledgements

Once again I thank my friend and colleague John Talbot for his beautiful diagrams and for his support. We make a great team and long may it continue! I also would like to thank Philips Medical Systems, Bill Faulkner and Mike Kean for the use of some of their images in this book. Thanks again to all my friends and family and especially to Toni, Adam, Ben and Madeleine and to family in the USA.

Dedication

This book is dedicated to my 'Dear Old Dad', Joe Barbieri.

Magnetism and electromagnetism

homogeneous
magnetic field

paramagnetic
substance

paramagnetic substance
in the magnetic field

Figure 1.1 Paramagnetic properties.

homogeneous
magnetic field

diamagnetic
substance

diamagnetic substance
in the magnetic field

Figure 1.2 Diamagnetic properties.

homogeneous
magnetic field

ferromagnetic
substance

ferromagnetic substance
in the magnetic field

Figure 1.3 Ferromagnetic properties.

magnetic
field in
direction
of fingers

current in direction
of thumb

conductor

Figure 1.4 The right-hand thumb rule.

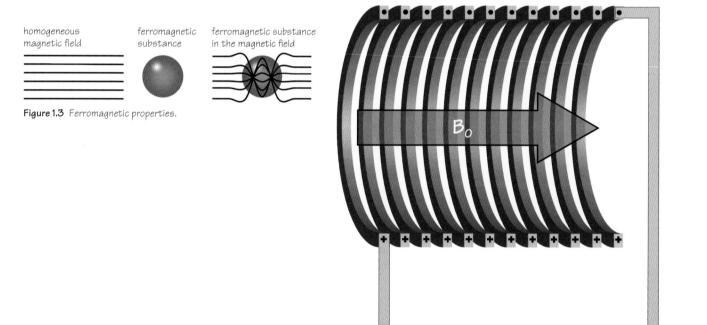

B_0

Figure 1.5 A simple electromagnet.

Magnetic susceptibility

The **magnetic susceptibility** of a substance is the ability of external magnetic fields to affect the nuclei of a particular atom, and is related to the electron configurations of that atom. The nucleus of an atom, which is surrounded by paired electrons, is more protected from, and unaffected by, the external magnetic field than the nucleus of an atom with unpaired electrons. There are three types of magnetic susceptibility: **paramagnetism**, **diamagnetism** and **ferromagnetism**.

Paramagnetism

Paramagnetic substances contain unpaired electrons within the atom that induce a small magnetic field about themselves known as the **magnetic moment**. With no external magnetic field these magnetic moments occur in a random pattern and cancel each other out. In the presence of an external magnetic field, paramagnetic substances align with the direction of the field and so the magnetic moments add together. Paramagnetic substances affect external magnetic fields in a positive way, resulting in a local increase in the magnetic field (Figure 1.1). An example of a paramagnetic substance is oxygen.

Diamagnetism

With no external magnetic field present, diamagnetic substances show no net magnetic moment as the electron currents caused by their motions add to zero.

When an external magnetic field is applied, diamagnetic substances show a small magnetic moment that opposes the applied field. Substances of this type are therefore slightly repelled by the magnetic field and have negative magnetic susceptibilities (Figure 1.2). Examples of diamagnetic substances include water and inert gasses.

Ferromagnetism

When a ferromagnetic substance comes into contact with a magnetic field, the results are strong attraction and alignment. They retain their magnetization even when the external magnetic field has been removed. Ferromagnetic substances remain magnetic, are permanently magnetized and subsequently become permanent magnets. An example of a ferromagnetic substance is iron.

Magnets are **bipolar** as they have two poles, north and south. The magnetic field exerted by them produces magnetic field lines or lines of force running from the magnetic south to the north poles of the magnet (Figure 1.3). They are called **magnetic lines of flux**. The number of lines per unit area is called the **magnetic flux density**. The strength of the magnetic field, expressed by the notation (B) – or, in the case of more than one field, the primary field (B_0) and the secondary field (B_1) – is measured in one of three units: **gauss (G)**, **kilogauss (kG)** and **tesla (T)**. If two magnets are brought close together, there are forces of attraction and repulsion between them depending on the orientation of their poles relative to each other. Like poles repel and opposite poles attract.

Electromagnetism

Magnetic fields are generated by moving charges (electrical current). The direction of the magnetic field can either be clockwise or counterclockwise with respect to the direction of flow of the current. **Ampere's law** or **Fleming's right-hand rule** determines the magnitude and direction of the magnetic field due to a current; if you point your right thumb along the direction of the current, then the magnetic field points along the direction of the curled fingers (Figure 1.4).

Just as moving electrical charge generates magnetic fields, changing magnetic fields generate electric currents. When a magnet is moved in and out of a closed circuit, an oscillating current is produced which ceases the moment the magnet stops moving. Such a current is called an **induced electric current** (Figure 1.5).

Faraday's law of induction explains the phenomenon of an induced current. The change of magnetic flux through a closed circuit induces an **electromotive force (emf)** in the circuit. The emf drives a current in the circuit and is the result of a changing magnetic field inducing an electric field.

The laws of electromagnetic induction (Faraday) state that the induced emf:

(1) is proportional to the rate of change of magnetic field and the area of the circuit;

(2) is in a direction so that it opposes the change in magnetic field which causes it (**Lenz's law**).

Electromagnetic induction is a basic physical phenomenon of MRI but is specifically involved in the following:

• the spinning charge of a hydrogen proton causes a magnetic field to be induced around it (see Chapter 2).

• the movement of the **net magnetization vector (NMV)** across the area of a receiver coil induces an electrical charge in the coil (see Chapter 4).

2 Atomic structure

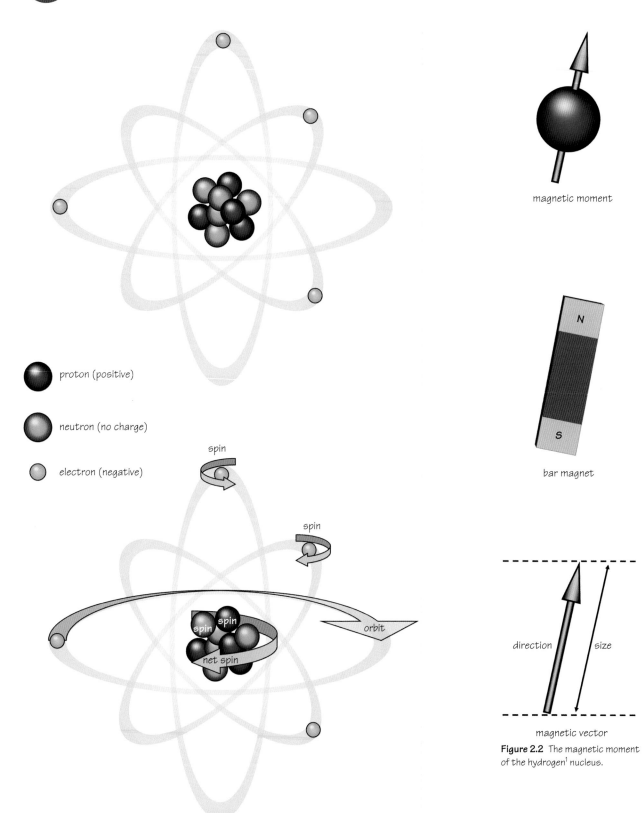

proton (positive)

neutron (no charge)

electron (negative)

Figure 2.1 The atom.

magnetic moment

bar magnet

magnetic vector

Figure 2.2 The magnetic moment of the hydrogen[1] nucleus.

Introduction

The atom consists of the following particles:

Protons
- in the nucleus
- are positively charged

Neutrons
- in the nucleus
- have no charge

Electrons
- orbit the nucleus
- are negatively charged (Figure 2.1).

The following terms are used to characterize an atom:

Atomic number: number of protons in the nucleus and determines the type of element the atoms make up.

Mass number: sum of the neutrons and protons in the nucleus.

Atoms of the same element having a different mass number are called **isotopes**.

In a stable atom the number of negatively charged electrons equals the number of positively charged protons. Atoms with a deficit or excess number of electrons are called **ions**.

Motion within the atom

- Negatively charged electrons spinning on their own axis.
- Negatively charged electrons orbiting the nucleus.
- Particles within the nucleus spinning on their own axes (Figure 2.1).

Each type of motion produces a magnetic field (see Chapter 1). In MR we are concerned with the motion of particles within the nucleus and the nucleus itself.

MR active nuclei

Protons and neutrons spin about their own axis within the nucleus. The direction of spin is random so that some particles spin clockwise, and others anticlockwise.

When a nucleus has an **even mass number** the spins cancel each other out so the nucleus has **no net spin**.

When a nucleus has an **odd mass number**, the spins do not cancel each other out and the **nucleus spins**.

As protons have charge, a nucleus with an odd mass number has a net charge as well as a net spin. Due to the laws of electromagnetic induction (see Chapter 1), a moving unbalanced charge induces a magnetic field around itself. The direction and size of the magnetic field is denoted by a magnetic moment or arrow (Figure 2.2). The total magnetic moment of the nucleus is the vector sum of all the magnetic moments of protons in the nucleus. The length of the arrow represents the magnitude of the magnetic moment. The direction of the arrow denotes the direction of alignment of the magnetic moment.

Nuclei with an odd number of protons are said to be **MR active**. They act like tiny bar magnets. There are many types of elements that are MR active. They all have an odd mass number. The common MR active nuclei, together with their mass numbers, are:

hydrogen 1   carbon 13   nitrogen   15   oxygen 17
fluorine 19   sodium 23   phosphorus 31

The isotope of hydrogen called **protium** is the MR active nucleus used in MRI as it has a mass and atomic number of 1. The nucleus of this isotope consists of a single proton and has no neutrons. It is used for MR imaging because:

- it is abundant in the human body (e.g. in fat and water);
- its solitary proton gives it a relatively large magnetic moment.

3 Alignment and precession

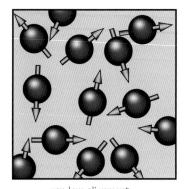

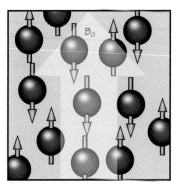

random alignment
no external field

alignment
external magnetic field

Figure 3.1 Alignment: classical theory.

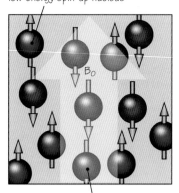

low-energy spin-up nucleus

high-energy spin-down nucleus

Figure 3.2 Alignment: quantum theory.

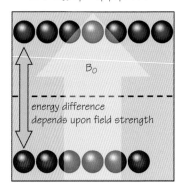

low-energy spin-up population

energy difference
depends upon field strength

high-energy spin-down population

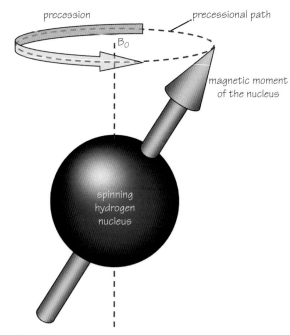

procession

precessional path

magnetic moment
of the nucleus

spinning
hydrogen
nucleus

Figure 3.3 Precession.

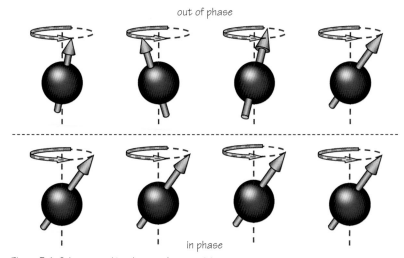

out of phase

in phase

Figure 3.4 Coherent and incoherent phase positions.

Alignment

In a normal environment the magnetic moments of MR active nuclei point in a random direction, and produce no overall magnetic effect. When nuclei are placed in an external magnetic field their magnetic moments line up with the magnetic field flux lines. This is called **alignment**. Alignment is described using two theories.

The classical theory (Figure 3.1)

This uses the direction of the magnetic moments to illustrate alignment.

• **Parallel alignment:** alignment of magnetic moments in the *same* direction as the main field.

• **Anti-parallel alignment:** alignment of magnetic moments in the *opposite* direction to the main field.

At room temperature there are always more nuclei with their magnetic moments aligned parallel than anti-parallel. The net magnetism of the patient (termed the **net magnetization vector**; **NMV**) is therefore aligned parallel to the main field.

The quantum theory (Figure 3.2)

This uses the energy level of the nuclei to illustrate alignment. According to the quantum theory, magnetic moments of hydrogen nuclei align in the presence of an external magnetic field in two energy states.

• **Spin-up** nuclei have low energy and do not have enough energy to oppose the main field. These are nuclei that align their magnetic moments parallel to the main field in the classical description.

• **Spin-down** nuclei have high energy and have enough energy to oppose the main field. These are nuclei that align their magnetic moments anti-parallel to the main field in the classical description.

The magnetic moments of the nuclei actually align at an angle to B_0 due to the force of repulsion between B_0 and the magnetic moments.

What do the quantum and classical theories tell us?

• Hydrogen only has two energy states – high or low. Therefore the magnetic moments of hydrogen only align in the parallel or anti-parallel directions. **The magnetic moments of hydrogen cannot orientate themselves in any other direction.**

• The patient's temperature is an important factor that determines whether a nucleus is in the high or low energy population. In clinical imaging, thermal effects are discounted as we assume the patient's temperature is the same inside and outside the magnetic field (thermal equilibrium).

• The magnetic moments of hydrogen are constantly changing their orientation because nuclei are constantly moving between high and low energy states. The nuclei gain and lose energy from B_0 and their magnetic moments are constantly altering their alignment relative to B_0.

• In thermal equilibrium, at any moment there are a greater proportion of nuclei with their magnetic moments aligned with the field than against it. This excess aligned with B_0 produces a net magnetic effect called the NMV that aligns with the main magnetic field.

• As the magnitude of the external magnetic field increases, more magnetic moments line up in the parallel direction because the amount of energy they must possess to oppose the stronger field and line up anti-parallel is increased. As the field strength increases, the low-energy population increases and the high-energy population decreases. As a result the NMV increases.

Precession

Every MR active nucleus is spinning on its own axis. Due to the influence of the external magnetic field these nuclei produce a secondary spin (Figure 3.3). This spin is called **precession** and causes the magnetic moments of MR active nuclei to describe a circular path around B_0. The speed at which the magnetic moments spin about the external magnetic field is called the **precessional frequency**.

The **Larmor equation** is used to calculate the frequency or speed of precession for a specific nucleus in a specific magnetic field strength. The Larmor equation is stated as follows:

$$\omega_0 = B_0 \times \lambda$$

• The precessional frequency is denoted by ω_0

• The strength of the external field is expressed in tesla (T) and denoted by the symbol B_0

• The **gyromagnetic ratio** is the precessional frequency of a specific nucleus at 1T and has units of MHz/T. It is denoted by the Greek symbol lambda (λ). As it is a constant of proportionality the precessional frequency is proportional to the strength of the external field.

The precessional frequencies of hydrogen (gyromagnetic ratio 42.57 MHz/T) commonly found in clinical MRI are:

• 21.285 MHz at 0.5 T
• 42.57 MHz at 1 T
• 63.86 MHz at 1.5 T

The precessional frequency corresponds to the range of frequencies in the electromagnetic spectrum of **radiowaves**. Therefore hydrogen precesses at a low frequency. At equilibrium the magnetic moments of the nuclei are out of phase with each other. **Phase** refers to the position of the magnetic moments on their precessional path.

• **Out of phase** or **incoherent** means that the magnetic moments of hydrogen are at different places on the precessional path.

• **In phase** or **coherent** means that the magnetic moments of hydrogen are at the same place on the precessional path (Figure 3.4).

4 Resonance and signal generation

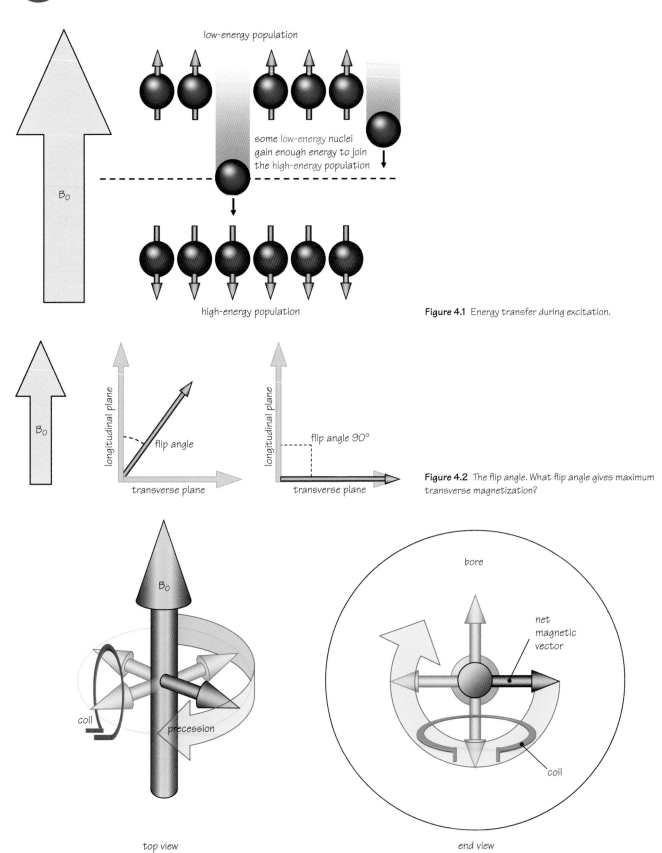

low-energy population

some low-energy nuclei gain enough energy to join the high-energy population

high-energy population

Figure 4.1 Energy transfer during excitation.

B_0

longitudinal plane

flip angle

transverse plane

longitudinal plane

flip angle 90°

transverse plane

Figure 4.2 The flip angle. What flip angle gives maximum transverse magnetization?

B_0

coil

precession

bore

net magnetic vector

coil

top view

end view

Figure 4.3 Generation of the MR signal. Why would you expect the MR signal to be alternating?

Resonance

Resonance is an energy transition that occurs when an object is subjected to a frequency the same as its own. In MR, resonance is induced by applying a **radiofrequency (RF) pulse**:
- at the same frequency as the precessing hydrogen nuclei;
- at 90° to B_0.

This causes the hydrogen nuclei to resonate (receive energy from the RF pulse) whereas other types of MR active nuclei do not resonate. As their gyromagnetic ratios are different from that of hydrogen their precessional frequencies are also different to that of hydrogen. They will only resonate if RF at their specific precessional frequency is applied. As RF is only applied at the same frequency as the precessional frequency of hydrogen, only hydrogen nuclei resonate. The other types of MR active nuclei do not. Two things happen to the hydrogen nuclei at resonance: energy absorption and phase coherence.

Energy absorption

The hydrogen nuclei absorb energy from the RF pulse (excitation pulse). The absorption of applied RF energy at 90° to B_0 causes an increase in the number of high-energy, spin-down nuclei (Figure 4.1). If just the right amount of energy is applied the number of nuclei in the spin-up position equals the number in the spin-down position. As a result the NMV (which represents the balance between spin-up and spin-down nuclei) lies in a plane at 90° to the external field (the **transverse plane**) as the net magnetization lies between the two energy states. As the NMV has been moved through 90° from B_0, it has a **flip or tip angle** of 90° (Figure 4.2).

Phase coherence

The magnetic moments of the nuclei move into phase with each other (see Chapter 3). As the magnetic moments are in phase both in the spin-up and spin-down positions and the spin-up nuclei are in phase with the spin-down nuclei, the net effect is one of precession, so the NMV precesses in the transverse plane at the Larmor frequency.

Learning point

It is important to understand that when a patient is placed in the magnet and is scanned, hydrogen nuclei do not move. Nuclei are not flipped onto their sides in the transverse plane and neither are their magnetic moments. Only the magnetic moments of the nuclei move, aligning either with or against B_0. This is because hydrogen can only have two energy states, high or low (see Chapter 3). It is the NMV that lies in the transverse plane, *not* the magnetic moments, nor the nuclei themselves.

The MR signal

A receiver coil is situated in the transverse plane. As the NMV rotates around the transverse plane as a result of resonance, it passes across the receiver coil inducing a voltage in it (see Chapter 1). This voltage is the **MR signal** (Figure 4.3).

After a short period of time the RF pulse is removed. The signal induced in the receiver coil begins to decrease. This is because the in-phase component of the NMV in the transverse plane, which is passing across the receiver coil, begins to decrease as an increasingly higher proportion of spins become out of phase with each other. The amplitude of the voltage induced in the receiver coil therefore decreases. This is called **free induction decay** or **FID**:
- 'free' because of the absence of the RF pulse;
- 'induction decay' because of the decay of the induced signal in the receiver coil.

5 Contrast mechanisms

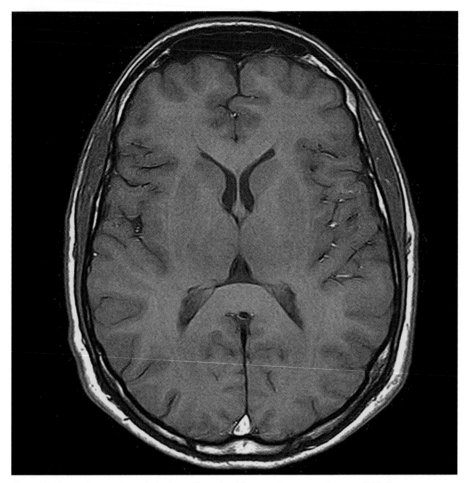

Figure 5.1 An axial image through the brain. Note the differences in contrast between CSF, fat, grey matter and white matter.

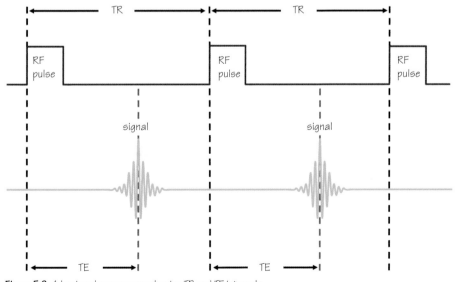

Figure 5.2 A basic pulse sequence showing TR and TE intervals.

What is contrast?

An image has contrast if there are areas of high signal (white on the image), as well as areas of low signal (dark on the image). Some areas have an intermediate signal (shades of grey, between white and black). The NMV can be separated into the individual vectors of the tissues present in the patient such as fat, cerebrospinal fluid (CSF), grey matter and white matter (Figure 5.1).

A tissue has a **high signal (white, hyperintense)** if it has a **large transverse component of magnetization** when the signal is measured. If there is a large component of transverse magnetization, the amplitude of the magnetization that cuts the coil is large, and the signal induced in the coil is also large.

A tissue has a **low signal (black, hypointense)**, if it has a **small transverse component of magnetization** when the signal is measured. If there is a small component of transverse magnetization, the amplitude of the magnetization that cuts the coil is small, and the signal induced in the coil is also small.

A tissue has an intermediate signal (grey, isointense), if it has a medium transverse component of magnetization when the signal is measured.

Image contrast is controlled by **extrinsic contrast parameters** (those that are controlled by the system operator). These include:

• **Repetition time (TR):** This is the time from the application of one RF pulse to the application of the next for a particular slice. It is measured in milliseconds (ms). The TR affects the length of a relaxation period in a particular slice after the application of one RF excitation pulse to the beginning of the next (see Chapter 7) (Figure 5.2).

• **Time to echo (TE):** This is the time between an RF excitation pulse and the collection of the signal. The TE affects the length of the relaxation period after the removal of an RF excitation pulse and the peak of the signal received in the receiver coil (see Chapter 8). It is also measured in ms (Figure 5.2);

• **Flip angle:** This is the angle through which the NMV is moved as a result of an RF excitation pulse (Figure 4.2);

• **Turbo-factor (TF)** or **echo train length (ETL)** (see Chapter 14);

• **Time from inversion (TI)** (see Chapter 16);

• **'b' value** (see Chapter 25).

Image contrast is also controlled by **intrinsic contrast mechanisms** (those that are inherent to the tissue and do not come under the operator's control). These include:

• T1 recovery time
• T2 decay time
• Proton density
• Flow
• Apparent diffusion coefficient (ADC).

The composition of fat and water

All substances possess molecules that are constantly in motion. This molecular motion is made up of rotational and transitional movements and is called **Brownian motion**. The faster the molecular motion, the more difficult it is for a substance to release energy to its surroundings.

• **Fat** comprises hydrogen atoms mainly linked to carbon, that make up large molecules. The large molecules in fat are closely packed together and have a slow rate of molecular motion due to inertia of the large molecules. They also have a low inherent energy which means they are able to absorb energy efficiently.

• **Water** comprises hydrogen atoms linked to oxygen. It consists of small molecules that are spaced far apart and have a high rate of molecular motion. They have a high inherent energy that means they are not able to absorb energy efficiently.

Because of these differences, tissues that contain fat and water produce different image contrast. This is because there are different **relaxation** rates in each tissue.

6 Relaxation mechanisms

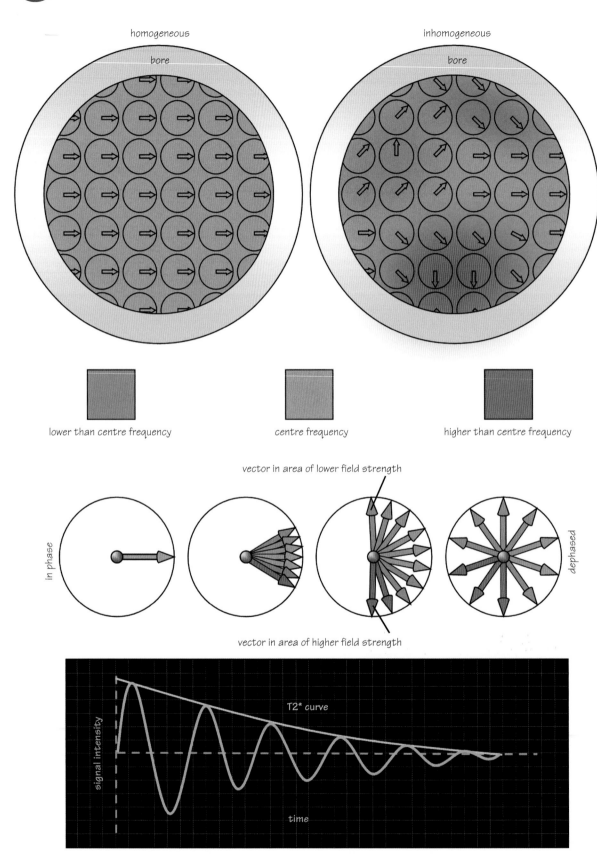

Figure 6.1 T2* decay and field inhomogeneities.

After the RF excitation pulse has been applied and resonance and the desired flip angle achieved, the RF pulse is removed. The signal induced in the receiver coil begins to decrease. This is because the coherent component of NMV in the transverse plane, which is passing across the receiver coil, begins to gradually decrease as an increasingly higher proportion of spins become out of phase with each other. The amplitude of the voltage induced in the receiver coil therefore gradually decreases. This is called **free induction decay** or **FID**. The NMV in the transverse plane decreases due to:
- relaxation processes;
- field inhomogeneities.

Relaxation processes

The magnetization in each tissue relaxes at different rates. This is one of the factors that create image contrast.

The withdrawal of the RF produces several effects:
- Nuclei emit energy absorbed from the RF pulse through a process known as **spin lattice energy transfer** and shift their magnetic moments from the high-energy state to the low-energy state. The NMV recovers and realigns to B_0. This relaxation process is called **T1 recovery**.
- Nuclei lose precessional coherence or dephase and the NMV decays in the transverse plane. The dephasing relaxation process is called **T2 decay**.

Nuclei lose their coherence in two ways:
- by the interactions of the intrinsic magnetic fields of adjacent nuclei (**spin-spin**) causing **T2 decay** (see Chapter 8);
- by **inhomogeneities** of the external magnetic field causing **T2* decay**.

Field inhomogeneities

Despite attempts to make the main magnetic field as uniform as possible, inhomogeneities of the external magnetic field are inevitable and slightly alter the magnitude of B_0, i.e. some small areas of the field have a magnetic field strength of slightly more or less than the main field strength.

Due to the Larmor equation, the precessional frequency of a spin is proportional to B_0 (see Chapter 3). Spins that pass through these inhomogeneities experience magnetic field strengths that are slightly different from B_0 and their precessional frequencies change. This results in a change in their phase and dephasing of the NMV (Figure 6.1). Due to a loss in phase coherence, transverse magnetization decays. This decay occurs exponentially and is known as **T2***. Magnetic field inhomogeneities cause the NMV to dephase before the intrinsic magnetic fields of nuclei can influence dephasing, i.e. T2* happens before T2. In order to produce images where T2 contrast can be visualized, ideally there must be a mechanism to rephase spins and compensate for magnetic field inhomogeneities. This is done by using **pulse sequences** (see Chapter 12).

7 T1 recovery

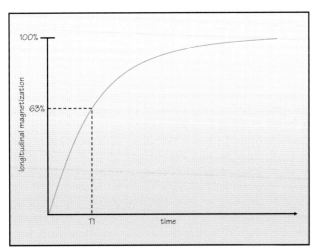

Figure 7.1 The T1 recovery curve.

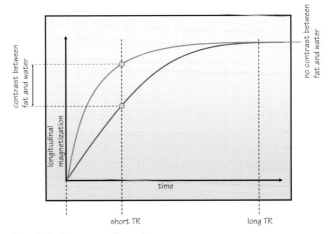

Figure 7.2 T1 recovery in fat and water.

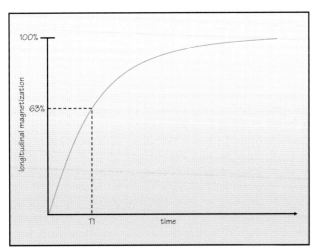

Figure 7.3 Saturation using a short TR.

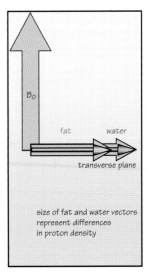

Figure 7.4 Non-saturation using a long TR.

T1 recovery is caused by the exchange of energy from nuclei to their surrounding environment or lattice. It is called **spin lattice energy transfer**. As the nuclei dissipate their energy their magnetic moments relax or return to B_0, i.e. they regain their longitudinal magnetization. The rate at which this occurs is an exponential process and occurs at different rates in different tissues.

The **T1 recovery time** of a particular tissue is an intrinsic contrast parameter that is inherent to the tissue being imaged. It is a constant for a particular tissue and is defined as the time it takes for 63% of the longitudinal magnetization to recover in that tissue (Figure 7.1). The period of time during which this occurs is the time between one excitation pulse and the next or the **TR** (see Chapter 5). The TR therefore determines how much T1 recovery occurs in a particular tissue.

T1 recovery in fat (Figure 7.2)

• T1 relaxation occurs as a result of nuclei exchanging the energy given to them by the RF pulse to their surrounding environment. The efficiency of this process determines the T1 recovery time of the tissue in which they are situated.

• Due to the fact that fat is able to absorb energy quickly (see Chapter 5), **the T1 recovery time of fat is very short**, i.e. nuclei dispose of their energy to the surrounding fat tissue and return to B_0 in a short time.

T1 recovery in water (Figure 7.2)

• Water is very inefficient at receiving energy from nuclei (see Chapter 5). **The T1 recovery time of water is therefore quite long**, i.e. nuclei take a lot longer to dispose of their energy to the surrounding water tissue and return to B_0.

• In addition, the efficiency of spin lattice energy transfer depends on how closely molecular motion of the molecules matches the Larmor frequency. If there is a good match between the rate of molecular tumbling and the precessional frequency of spins, energy can be efficiently exchanged between hydrogen and the surrounding molecular lattice.

• The Larmor frequency is relatively slow and therefore fat is much better at this type of energy exchange than water, whose molecular motion is much faster than the Larmor frequency (see Chapter 5). This is another reason why **fat has a shorter T1 recovery time than water**.

Control of T1 recovery

The TR controls how much of the NMV in fat or water has recovered before the application of the next RF pulse.

Short TRs do not permit full longitudinal recovery in most tissues so that there are different longitudinal components in fat and water. These different longitudinal components are converted to different transverse components after the next excitation pulse has been applied. As the NMV does not recover completely to the positive longitudinal axis, they are pushed beyond the transverse plane by the succeeding 90° RF pulse. This is called **saturation**. When saturation occurs there is a contrast difference between fat and water due to differences in their T1 recovery times (Figure 7.3).

Long TRs allow full recovery of the longitudinal components in most tissues. There is no difference in the magnitude of their longitudinal components. There is no contrast difference between fat and water due to differences in T1 recovery times when using long TRs. Any differences seen in contrast are due to differences in the number of protons or **proton density** of each tissue. The proton density of a particular tissue is an intrinsic contrast parameter and is therefore inherent to the tissue being imaged (Figure 7.4).

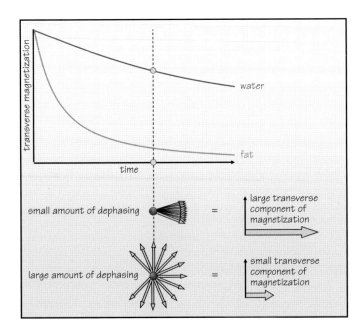

Figure 8.1 T2 contrast generation.

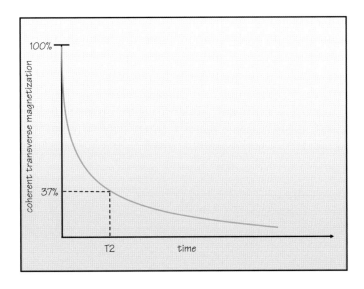

Figure 8.2 The T2 decay curve.

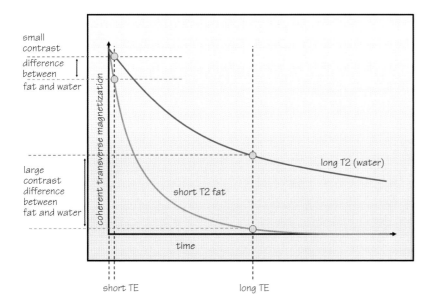

small contrast difference between fat and water

large contrast difference between fat and water

coherent transverse magnetization

long T2 (water)

short T2 fat

time

short TE   long TE

Figure 8.3 T2 decay in fat and water.

T2 decay is caused by the interaction between the magnetic fields of neighbouring spins. It is called **spin-spin**. It occurs as a result of the intrinsic magnetic fields of the nuclei interacting with each other. This produces a loss of phase coherence or dephasing, and results in decay of the NMV in the transverse plane. It is an exponential process and occurs at different rates in different tissues (Figure 8.1).

The **T2 decay time** of a particular tissue is an intrinsic contrast parameter and is inherent to the tissue being imaged. It is the time it takes for 63% of the transverse magnetization to be lost due to dephasing, i.e. transverse magnetization is reduced by 63% of its original value (37% remains) (Figure 8.2). The period of time during which this occurs is the time between the excitation pulse and the MR signal or the **TE** (see Chapter 5). The TE therefore determines how much T2 decay occurs in a particular tissue.

T2 decay in fat and water (Figure 8.3)
T2 relaxation occurs as a result of the spins of adjacent nuclei interacting with each other and exchanging energy. The efficiency of this process depends on how closely packed the molecules are to each other.

• In fat the molecules are more closely packed together than in water so that spin-spin is more efficient (see Chapter 5). **The T2 time of fat is therefore very short compared to that of water**.

• The **TE** controls how much transverse magnetization has been allowed to decay in fat and water when the signal is read.

Short TEs do not permit full dephasing in either fat or water, so their coherent transverse components are similar. There is little contrast difference between fat and water due to differences in T2 decay times using short TEs.

Long TEs allow dephasing of the transverse components in fat and water. There is a contrast difference between fat and water due to differences in T2 decay times when using long TEs.

It should be noted that fat and water represent the extremes in image contrast. Other tissues, such as muscle, grey matter and white matter have contrast characteristics that fall between fat and water.

9 T1 weighting

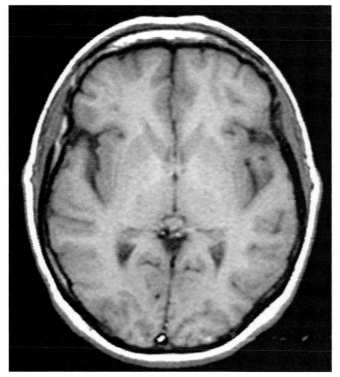

Figure 9.1 Axial T1 weighted image of the brain.

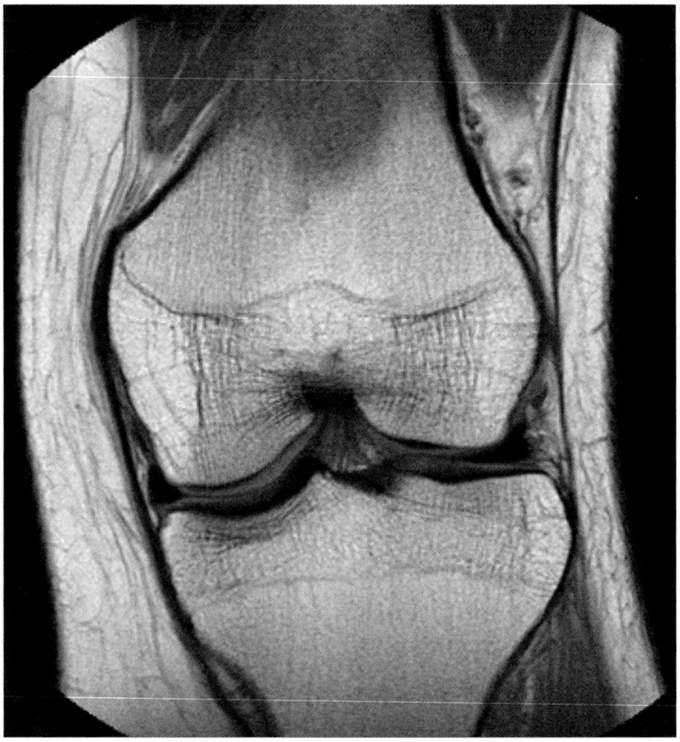

Figure 9.2 Coronal T1 weighted image of the knee.

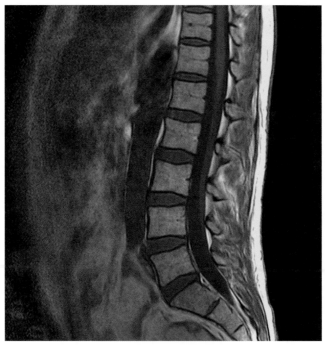

Figure 9.3 Sagittal T1 weighted image of the lumbar spine.

All intrinsic contrast mechanisms affect image contrast, regardless of the pulse sequence used. For example, tissues with a low proton density, and air, are always dark on an MR image and tissues in which nuclei move may be dark or bright depending on their velocity and the pulse sequence used (see Chapter 50).

In order to produce images where the contrast is predictable, parameters are selected to weight the image towards one contrast mechanism and away from the others. This achieved by understanding how extrinsic contrast parameters determine the degree to which intrinsic contrast parameters are allowed to affect image contrast. Extrinsic contrast parameters must be manipulated to accentuate one intrinsic contrast parameter and diminish the others. Flow and ADC effects are discussed later (see Chapters 25 and 50) and are not included in the following discussion. Proton density effects cannot be changed. T1 and T2 influences are manipulated by changing the TR and TE in the following way.

T1 weighting

In a **T1 weighted image**, differences in the T1 relaxation times of tissues must be accentuated and T2 effects must be reduced. To achieve this a TR is selected that is short enough to ensure that the NMV in neither fat nor water has had time to fully relax back to B_0 before the application of the next excitation pulse. The NMV in both fat and water is saturated (Figures 7.3 and 7.4). If the TR is long, the NMV in both fat and water recovers and their respective T1 relaxation times can no longer be distinguished (see Chapter 7).

• A T1 weighted image is an image whose contrast is predominantly due to the differences in T1 recovery times of tissues (Table 9.1).

• For T1 weighting, differences between the T1 times of tissues are exaggerated and to achieve this the TR must be short. At the same time, however, T2 effects must be minimized to avoid mixed weighting. To diminish T2 effects the TE must also be short.

• In T1 weighted images, tissues containing a high proportion of as fat, with short T1 relaxation times, are bright (high signal, hyperintense) because they recover most of their longitudinal magnetization during the short TR and therefore more magnetization is available to be flipped into the transverse plane by the next RF pulse and contribute to the signal.

• Tissues containing a high proportion of as water, with long T1 relaxation times, are dark (low signal, hypointense) because they do not recover much of their longitudinal magnetization during the short TR and therefore less magnetization is available to be flipped into the transverse plane by the next RF pulse and contribute to the signal.

• T1 weighted images best demonstrate anatomy but also show pathology if used after contrast enhancement (Figures 9.1, 9.2 and 9.3).

Typical values
• **TR:** 400–700 ms (shorter in gradient echo sequences)
• **TE:** 10–30 ms (shorter in gradient echo sequences)

Table 9.1 Signal intensities seen in T1 weighted images

High signal	Fat
	Haemangioma
	Intra-osseous lipoma
	Radiation change
	Degeneration fatty deposition
	Methaemoglobin
	Cysts with proteinaceous fluid
	Paramagnetic contrast agents
	Slow-flowing blood
Low signal	Cortical bone
	Avascular necrosis
	Infarction
	Infection
	Tumours
	Sclerosis
	Cysts
	Calcification
No signal	Air
	Fast-flowing blood
	Tendons
	Cortical bone
	Scar tissue
	Calcification

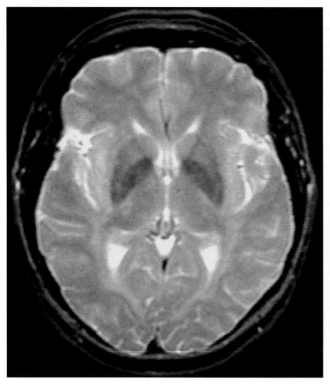

Figure 10.1 Axial T2 weighted image of the brain.

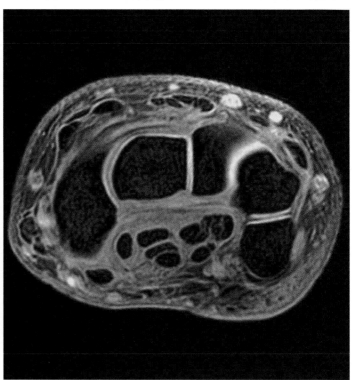

Figure 10.2 Axial T2 weighted image of the wrist.

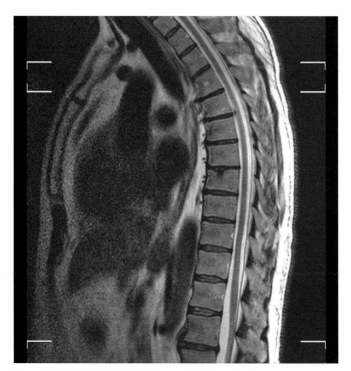

Figure 10.3 Sagittal T2 weighted image of the thoracic spine.

All intrinsic contrast parameters affect image contrast, regardless of the pulse sequence, TR and TE used. For example, tissues with a low proton density, and air, are always dark on an MR image, and tissues in which nuclei move may be dark or bright depending on their velocity and the pulse sequence used (see Chapter 50).

Therefore parameters are selected to weight the image towards one contrast mechanism and away from the others. This is achieved by understanding how extrinsic contrast parameters determine the degree to which intrinsic contrast parameters are allowed to affect image contrast. Extrinsic contrast parameters must be manipulated to accentuate one intrinsic contrast parameter and diminish the others. Flow and ADC effects are discussed later (see Chapters 25 and 50) and are not included in the following discussion. Proton density effects cannot be changed. T1 and T2 influences are manipulated by changing the TR and TE in the following way.

T2 weighting

In a **T2 weighted image** the differences in the T2 relaxation times of tissues must be demonstrated. To achieve this, a TE is selected that is long enough to ensure that the NMV in both fat and water has had time to decay. If the TE is too short, the NMV in neither fat nor water has had time to decay and their respective T2 times cannot be distinguished (Figure 8.3).

• A **T2 weighted image** is an image whose contrast is predominantly due to the differences in the T2 decay times of tissues (Table 10.1).

• For **T2 weighting** the differences between the T2 times of tissues are exaggerated, therefore the **TE** must be **long**. At the same time, however, T1 effects must be minimized to avoid mixed weighting. T1 effects are diminished by selecting a **long TR**.

• Tissues containing a high proportion of **fat**, with a short T2 decay time, are **dark** (low signal, hypointense) because they lose most of their coherent transverse magnetization during the TE period.

• Tissues containing a high proportion of **water**, with a long T2 decay time, are **bright** (high signal, hyperintense), because they retain most of their transverse coherence during the TE period.

• T2 weighted images best demonstrate pathology as most pathology has an increased water content and is therefore bright on T2 weighted images (Figures 10.1, 10.2 and 10.3).

Typical values
• **TR:** 2000+ ms (much shorter in gradient echo sequences)
• **TE:** 70+ ms (shorter in gradient echo sequences)

Table 10.1 Signal intensities seen in T2 weighted images

High signal	CSF
	Synovial fluid
	Haemangioma
	Infection
	Inflammation
	Oedema
	Some tumours
	Haemorrhage
	Slow-flowing blood
	Cysts
Low signal	Cortical bone
	Bone islands
	Deoxyhaemoglobin
	Haemosiderin
	Calcification
	T2 paramagnetic agents
No signal	Air
	Fast-flowing blood
	Tendons
	Cortical bone
	Scar tissue
	Calcification

11 Proton density weighting

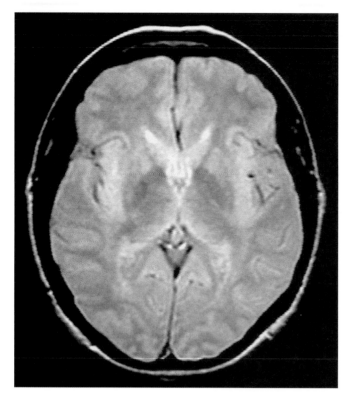

Figure 11.1 Axial proton density weighted image of the brain.

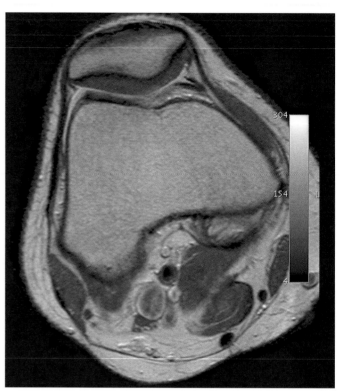

Figure 11.2 Axial proton density weighted image of the knee.

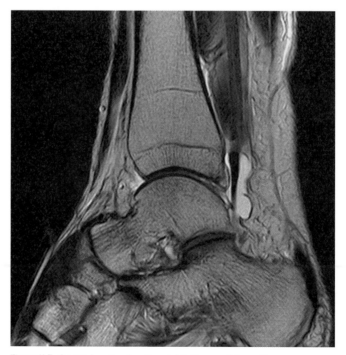

Figure 11.3 Sagittal proton density weighted image of the ankle.

All intrinsic contrast parameters affect image contrast regardless of the pulse sequence, TR and TE used. Therefore parameters are selected to **weight** the image towards one contrast mechanism and away from the others.

Proton density weighting

In a **proton density (PD) weighted image**, differences in the proton densities (number of hydrogen protons in the tissue) must be demonstrated. To achieve this both T1 and T2 effects are diminished. T1 effects are reduced by selecting a long TR and T2 effects are diminished by selecting a short TE (Figures 7.2 and 8.3).

• A **proton density weighted image** is an image whose contrast is predominantly due to differences in the proton density of the tissues (Table 11.1).

• Tissues with a **low proton density** are **dark** (low signal, hypointense) because the low number of protons results in a small component of transverse magnetization.

• Tissues with a **high proton density** are **bright** (high signal, hyperintense) because the high number of protons results in a large component of transverse magnetization.

• Cortical bone and air are always dark on MR images regardless of the weighting as they have a low proton density and therefore return little signal.

• Proton density weighted images show anatomy and some pathology (Figures 11.1, 11.2 and 11.3).

Typical values
• **TR:** 2000 ms+ (much shorter in gradient echo sequences)
• **TE:** 10–30 ms (shorter in gradient echo sequences)

Other types of weighting

Flow and the ADC of a tissue also affect weighting as they are intrinsic contrast mechanisms. Flow mechanisms are discussed in Chapter 50. Flow-related weighting is achieved in MR angiography techniques (see Chapters 51, 52 and 53). ADC-related weighting is achieved in diffusion weighting (see Chapter 25).

Table 11.1 Signal intensities seen in PD weighted images

High signal	CSF
	Synovial fluid
	Infection
	Inflammation
	Oedema
	Slow-flowing blood
	Cysts
	Fat
No or low signal	Air
	Fast-flowing blood
	Tendons
	Cortical bone
	Scar tissue
	Calcification

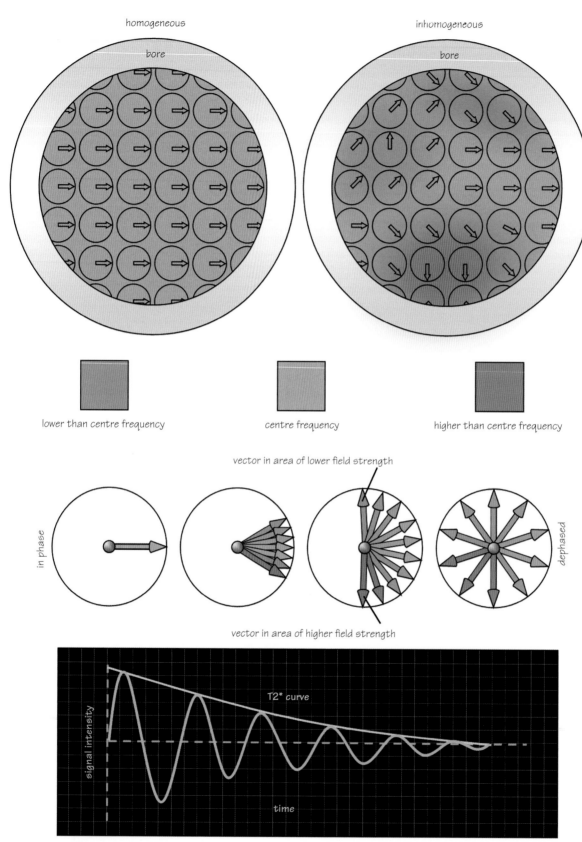

Figure 12.1 T2* decay and field inhomogeneities.

A **pulse sequence** is defined as a series of RF pulses, gradient applications and intervening time periods. They enable control of the way in which the system applies RF pulses and gradients. By selecting the intervening time periods, image weighting is controlled (see Chapter 5). Pulse sequences are required because, without a mechanism of refocusing spins, there is insufficient signal to produce an image. This is because dephasing occurs almost immediately after the RF excitation pulse has been removed.

Spins lose their phase coherence in two ways:
• by the interactions of the intrinsic magnetic fields of adjacent nuclei; **spin-spin** (T2) (see Chapter 6);
• by the **inhomogeneities** of the external magnetic field (T2*) (see Chapter 6).

Despite attempts to make the main magnetic field as uniform as possible via shimming (see Chapter 55), inhomogeneities of the external magnetic field are inevitable and slightly alter the magnitude of B_0, i.e. some small areas of the field have a magnetic field strength of slightly more or less than the main field strength.

Due to the Larmor equation, spins that pass through inhomogeneities experience a precessional frequency and phase change, and the resulting signal decays exponentially. It is called an FID and its rate of decay is termed **T2***. Magnetic field inhomogeneities cause the NMV to dephase before intrinsic magnetic fields of the nuclei can produce dephasing, i.e. T2* happens before T2 (see Chapter 6) (Figure 12.1).

The main purposes of pulse sequences are:
• to rephase spins and remove inhomogeneity effects and therefore produce a signal or echo that contains information about the T2 decay characteristics of tissue alone;
• to enable manipulation of the TE and TR to produce different types of contrast.

Spins are rephased in two ways (Table 12.1):
• by using a 180° RF pulse (used in all spin echo sequences);
• by using a gradient (used in all gradient echo sequences).

Table 12.1 Pulse sequences and their rephasing mechanisms

Use RF pulses to rephase spins	Use gradients to rephase spins
Spin echo	Gradient echo
Fast spin echo	Coherent gradient echo
Inversion recovery	Incoherent gradient echo
STIR	Steady-state free precession
FLAIR	Ultrafast sequences

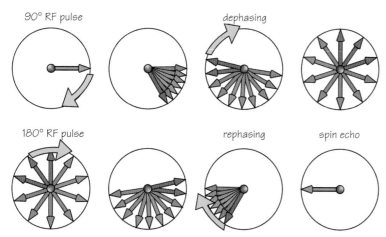

90° RF pulse   dephasing

180° RF pulse   rephasing   spin echo

Figure 13.1 180° RF rephasing.

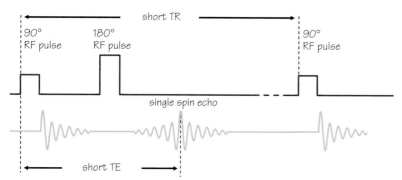

short TR

90° RF pulse   180° RF pulse   90° RF pulse

single spin echo

short TE

Figure 13.2 Single-echo spin echo sequence.

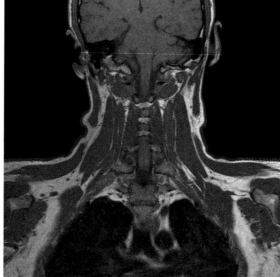

Figure 13.4 Coronal T1 SE sequence through the brachial plexus.

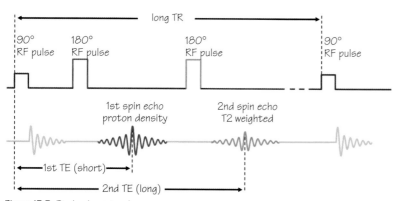

long TR

90° RF pulse   180° RF pulse   180° RF pulse   90° RF pulse

1st spin echo proton density   2nd spin echo T2 weighted

1st TE (short)

2nd TE (long)

Figure 13.3 Dual-echo spin echo sequence.

Conventional spin-echo (SE or CSE) pulse sequences are used to produce T1, T2 or proton density weighted images and are one the most basic pulse sequences used in MRI. In a spin-echo pulse sequence there is a 90° excitation pulse followed by a 180° rephasing pulse followed by an **echo**.

Mechanisms

• After the application of the 90° RF pulse, spins lose precessional coherence because of an increase or decrease in their precessional frequency caused by the magnetic field inhomogeneities. This results in a decay of coherent magnetization in the transverse plane and the ability to generate a signal is lost (see Chapter 6).

• Spins that experience an increase in precessional frequency gain phase relative to those that experience a decrease in precessional frequency who lag behind. Dephasing can be imagined as a 'fan' where spins that lag behind precess more slowly, and those that gain phase precess more quickly.

• A 180° RF pulse flips magnetic moments of the dephased spins through 180°. The fast edge of the fan is now positioned behind the slow edge. The fast edge eventually catches up with the slow edge, therefore rephasing the spins. This is called **rephasing** (Figure 13.1).

• The coherent signal in the receiver coil is regenerated and can be measured. This regenerated signal is called an **echo** and, because an RF pulse has been used to generate it, it is specifically called a **spin echo**.

• Rephasing the spins eliminates the effect of the magnetic field inhomogeneities. Whenever a 180° RF rephasing pulse is applied, a spin echo results. Rephasing pulses may be applied either once or several times to produce either one or several spin echoes.

Contrast

CSE is usually used in one of two ways:

A **single spin echo** pulse consists of a single 180° RF pulse applied after the excitation pulse to produce a single spin echo (Figure 13.2). This a typical sequence used to produce a T1 weighted set of images.

• The **TR** is the length of time from one 90° RF pulse to the next 90° RF pulse in a particular slice. For T1 weighted imaging a short TR is used.

• The **TE** is the length of time from the 90° RF pulse to the midpoint or peak of the signal generated after the 180° RF pulse, i.e. the spin echo. For T1 weighted imaging a short TE is used.

A **dual echo sequence** consists of two 180° pulses applied to produce two spin echoes. This is a sequence that provides two images per slice location: one that is proton density weighted and one that is T2 weighted (Figure 13.3).

• The first echo has a short TE and a long TR and results in a set of proton density weighted images.

• The second echo has a long TE and a long TR and results in a T2 weighted set of images. This echo has less amplitude than the first echo because more T2 decay has occurred by this point.

Typical values

Single echo (for T1 weighting)
• **TR:** 400–700 ms
• **TE:** 10–30 ms

Dual echo (for PD/T2 weighting)
• **TR:** 2000+ ms
• **TE1:** 20 ms
• **TE2:** 80 ms

Uses

Spin echo sequences are still considered the 'gold standard' (Table 13.1) in that the contrast they produce is understood and is predictable. They produce T1, T2 and PD weighted images of good quality and may be used in any part of the body, for any indication (Figure 13.4).

Table 13.1 Advantages and disadvantage of conventional spin echo

Advantages	Disadvantage
Good image quality	Long scan times
Very versatile	
True T2 weighting	
Available on all systems	
Gold standard for image contrast and weighting	

14 Fast or turbo spin echo – how it works

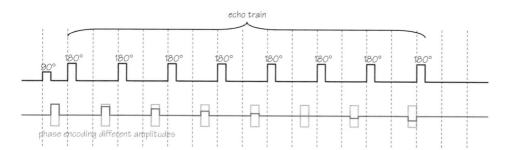

Figure 14.1 The echo train in TSE.

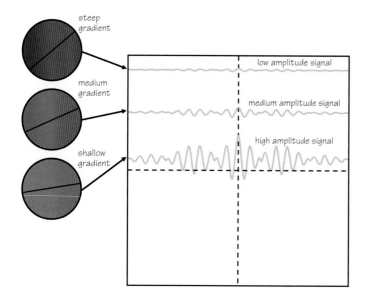

Figure 14.2 Phase encoding versus signal amplitude.

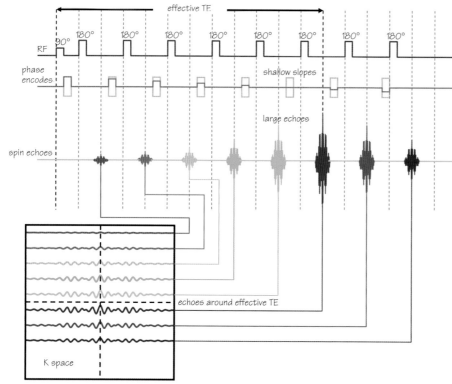

Figure 14.3 K space filling and phase reordering.

Fast or turbo spin echo (FSE or TSE) is a much faster version of conventional spin echo. In spin echo sequences, one phase encoding only is performed during each TR (see Chapter 32). The scan time is a function of TR, NSA and phase matrix (see Chapter 43). One of the ways of speeding up a conventional sequence is to reduce the number of phase-encoding steps. However, this normally results in a loss of resolution (see Chapter 42). TSE overcomes this by still performing the same number of phase encodings, thereby maintaining phase resolution, but more than one phase encoding is performed per TR, reducing the scan time.

Mechanism

• TSE employs a train of 180° rephasing pulses, each one producing a spin echo. This train of spin echoes is called an **echo train**. The number of 180° RF pulses and resultant echoes is called the **echo train length (ETL)** or **turbo factor**. The spacing between each echo is called the **echo spacing**.

• After each rephasing, a phase-encoding step is performed and data from the resultant echo is stored in K space (see Chapter 32) (Figure 14.1). Therefore several lines of K space are filled every TR instead of one line as in conventional spin echo. As K space is filled more rapidly, the scan time decreases.

• Typically 2 to 24 180° RF pulses are applied during every TR, although many more can be applied if required. As several phase encodings are also performed during each TR, the scan time is reduced. For example, if a factor of 16 has been used, 16 phase encodings are performed per TR and therefore 16 lines of K space are filled per TR instead of 1 as in conventional spin echo. Therefore the scan time is 1/16 of the original scan time (Table 14.1). The **higher** the turbo factor the **shorter** the scan time.

Contrast

• Each echo has a different TE and data from each echo is used to produce one image – as opposed to dual echo CSE when two echoes have different TEs but produce two sets of images, one PD and the other T2. There would normally be a mixture of weighting.

• In any sequence, each phase encoding step applies a different slope of phase gradient to phase shift each slice by a different amount. This ensures that data is placed in a different line of K space.

• The very **steep** gradient slopes significantly **reduce the amplitude** of the resultant echo/signal because they reduce the rephasing effect of the 180° rephasing pulse. **Shallow** gradients, on the other hand, do not have this effect and the amplitude of the resultant **echo/signal is maximized** (see Chapter 33) (Figure 14.2).

• When the TE is selected (known as the **effective TE** in TSE sequences) the resultant image must have a weighting corresponding to that TE, i.e. if the TE is set at 102 ms a T2 weighted image is obtained (assuming the TR is long).

• The system therefore orders the phase encodings so that those that produce the most signal (the shallowest ones) are used on echoes produced from 180° pulses nearest to the effective TE selected. The steepest gradients (which reduce the signal) are reserved for those echoes that are produced by 180° pulses furthest away from the effective TE. Therefore the resultant image is mostly made from data acquired at approximately the correct TE, although some other data is present (Figure 14.3).

Table 14.1 TSE time-saving illustrations

Pulse sequence	Scan time
SE, 256 phase encodings, 1NSA	$256 \times 1 \times TR = 256 \times TR$
TSE, 256 phase encodings, 1 NSA and ETL 16	$256 \times 1 \times TR/16 = 16 \times TR$

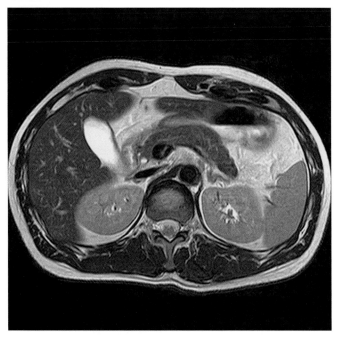

Figure 15.1 Axial T2 weighted TSE image of the abdomen.

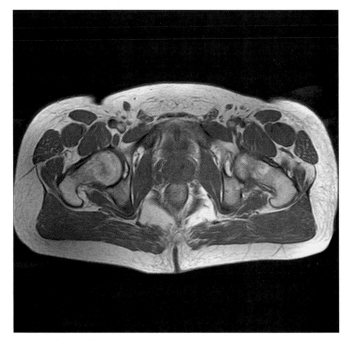

Figure 15.2 Axial T1 weighted TSE image of the male pelvis.

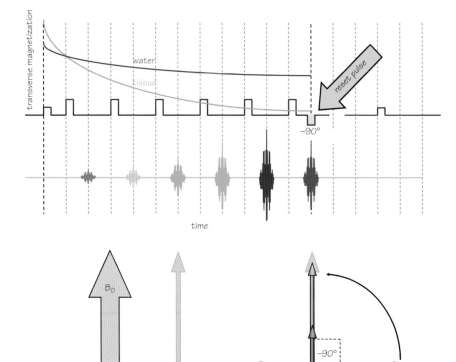

Figure 15.3 The fast recovery or 'drive' sequence.

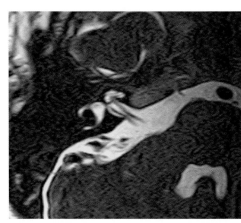

Figure 15.4 Fast recovery or 'drive' image of the internal auditory meatus.

Due to different contrasts being present in the image, the contrast of TSE is unique:

• In T2 weighted scans, water and fat are hyperintense (bright). This is because the succession of 180° RF pulses reduces the spin-spin interactions in fat, thereby increasing its T2 decay time (**J coupling**). Techniques used to suppress fat signal are therefore sometimes required to differentiate fat and pathology in T2 weighted TSE sequences.

• Muscle is often darker than in conventional spin echo T2 weighted images. This is because the succession of RF pulses increases **magnetization transfer** effects that produce saturation (see Chapter 41).

• In T1 weighted imaging, CNR is sometimes reduced so that the images look rather 'flat'. It is therefore best used when inherent contrast is good.

Typical values
Dual echo
• **TR:** 2500–8000 ms (for slice number)
• **Effective TE1:** 17 ms
• **Effective TE2:** 102 ms
• **Turbo factor 8:** this may be split so that the PD image is acquired with the first four echoes and the T2 with the second four echoes.

Single echo T2 weighting
• **TR:** 4000–8000 ms
• **TE:** 102 ms
• **Turbo factor:** 16

Single echo T1 weighting
• **TR:** 600 ms
• **TE:** 10 ms
• **Turbo factor:** 4

Uses
TSE produces T1, T2 or proton density scans in a fraction of the time of CSE (Figures 15.1 and 15.2). Due to the fact that the scan times are reduced, matrix size can be increased to improve spatial resolution. TSE is usually used in the brain, spine, joints, extremities and the pelvis. As TSE is incompatible with phase-reordered respiratory compensation techniques, it can only be used in the chest and abdomen with respiratory triggering, breath-hold or multiple NSA.

Systems that have sufficiently powerful gradients can use TSE in a single-shot mode (see Chapter 39), or via a slightly slower version called multi-shot. Both of these techniques permit image acquisition in a single breath-hold. In addition, using very long TEs and TRs permits very heavy T2 weighting (**watergrams**). Table 15.1 lists some advantages and disadvantages of TSE.

A modification of TSE that is sometimes called **fast recovery** or **drive** adds an additional 'reset' pulse at the end of the TR period. This pulse 'drives' any residual magnetization in the transverse plane at the end of each TR back into the longitudinal plane (Figure 15.3). This is then available to be flipped into the transverse plane by the next excitation pulse. This sequence provides a high signal intensity in water even when using a short TR and therefore short scan time (Figure 15.4). This is because water has a long T2 decay time; therefore tissue with high water content has residual transverse magnetization at the end of each TR. Hence this is the main tissue that is driven back up to the longitudinal plane by the reset pulse and is therefore the dominant tissue in terms of signal.

Table 15.1 Advantages and disadvantages of TSE

Advantages	Disadvantages
Short scan times	Some flow artefacts increased
High-resolution imaging	Incompatible with some imaging options
Increased T2 weighting	Some contrast interpretation problems
Magnetic susceptibility decreases*	Image blurring possible

*Also a disadvantage, e.g. haemorrhage not detected/delineated.

16 Inversion recovery

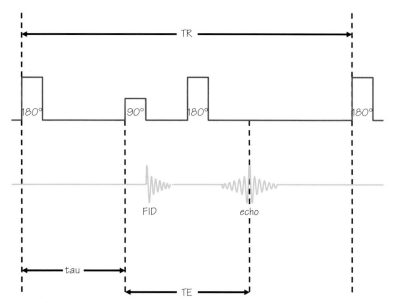

Figure 16.1 The inversion recovery sequence.

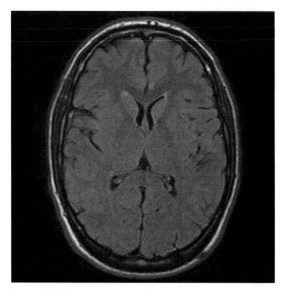

Figure 16.3 Axial FLAIR image of the brain.

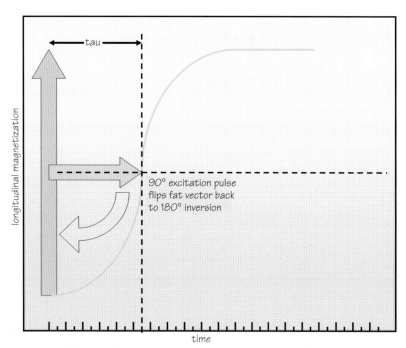

90° excitation pulse
flips fat vector back
to 180° inversion

Figure 16.2 How the use of short TI suppresses the signal from fat in a STIR sequence.

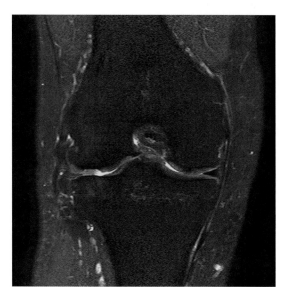

Figure 16.4 Coronal STIR image of the knee.

Inversion recovery (IR) sequences were initially designed to produce very heavy T1 weighting. However at present they are mainly used in conjunction with a TSE sequence to produce T2 weighted images in which certain tissues are suppressed. Both are described here.

Mechanism

- Inversion recovery is a spin echo sequence that begins with a 180° inverting pulse. This inverts the NMV through 180°. The TR is the time between successive 180° inverting pulses for a particular slice.
- When the pulse is removed the NMV begins to relax back to B_0. A 90° pulse is then applied at time interval TI (time from inversion) after the 180° inverting pulse.
- A further 180° RF pulse is applied which rephases spins in the transverse plane and produces an echo at time TE after the excitation pulse (Figure 16.1).

Contrast

- The TI is the main factor that controls weighting in IR sequences. If the TI is sufficiently long enough to allow the NMV to pass through the transverse plane, the contrast depends on the degree of saturation that is produced by the 90° pulse (as in spin echo), i.e. if the 90° pulse is applied shortly after the NMV has passed through the transverse plane, heavy saturation and T1 weighting results. TIs of 300–700 ms result in this type of heavy T1 weighting. Certain TI values result in suppression of signal from tissues.
- The TE controls the amount of T2 decay. For T1 weighting it must be short, for T2 weighting, long.
- The TR must always be long enough to allow full longitudinal recovery of magnetization before each inverting pulse. As result, traditional inversion recovery sequences are associated with a very long TR and therefore long scan time.

Fast inversion recovery is a combination of inversion recovery and turbo spin echo. In this sequence the NMV is flipped through 180° into full saturation by a 180° inverting pulse. As in conventional inversion recovery, the TR is the time between each successive 180° pulse in a particular slice. At a time TI, the 90° excitation pulse is applied. However after this, multiple 180° rephasing pulses are applied to produce multiple echoes that are phase encoded with a different slope of gradient. As in turbo spin echo, multiple lines of K space are filled each TR, thereby significantly reducing the scan time. This modification of inversion recovery is now used in preference to the conventional sequence because, as the TR required for IR sequences must be increased in order to permit full recovery of the longitudinal magnetization, scan times are very long. Fast IR allows much shorter scan times to be implemented. The parameters used are similar to conventional IR except that the ETL or turbo factor must be selected. This should be short for T1 weighting and long for T2 weighting.

With both sequence types a further modification of the TI allows suppression of signal from various tissue types.

STIR (short TI inversion recovery) uses short TIs such as 100–180 ms depending on field strength. TIs of this magnitude place the 90° excitation pulse at the time that NMV of fat is passing exactly through the transverse plane. At this point (called the **null point**) there is no longitudinal component in fat. Therefore the 90° excitation pulse produces no transverse component in fat and therefore no signal. In this way a fat-suppressed image results (Figure 16.2).

FLAIR (fluid attenuated inversion recovery) uses long TIs such as 1700–2200 ms depending on field strength to null the signal from CSF in exactly the same way as the STIR sequence. Because CSF has a long T1 recovery time, the TI must be longer to correspond with its null point.

Typical values

The required TI depends on the field strength (higher at higher fields).

T1 weighting
- **TI:** 300–700 ms
- **TE:** 10–20 ms
- **TR:** 2500+ ms
- **Turbo factor:** 4

STIR
- **TI:** 100–180 ms
- **TE:** 70+ ms (for T2 weighting)
- **TR:** 2500+ ms
- **Turbo factor:** 16

FLAIR
- **TI:** 1500–2200 ms
- **TE:** 70+ ms (for T2 weighting)
- **TR:** 2500+ ms
- **Turbo factor:** 12–16

Uses

Inversion recovery is a very versatile sequence (Table 16.1) that is mainly used in the CNS (T1 and FLAIR) and musculoskeletal systems (STIR). The FLAIR sequence increases the conspicuity of periventricular lesions such as MS plaques and lesions in the cervical and thoracic cord (Figure 16.3). STIR sequences are often called 'search and destroy' sequences when used in the musculoskeletal system as they null the signal from normal marrow, thereby increasing the conspicuity of bone lesions (Figure 16.4).

Table 16.1 Advantages and disadvantage of inversion recovery

Advantages	Disadvantage
Versatile	Long scan times (conventional IR)
Good image quality	
Sensitive to pathology	

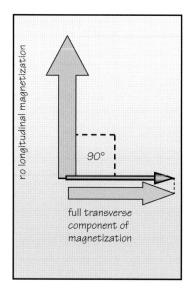
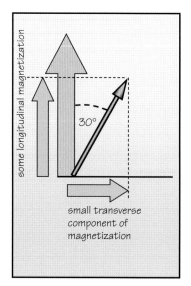

Figure 17.1 Flip angle versus signal amplitude.

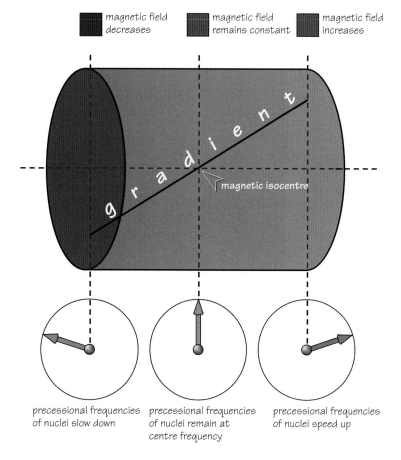

Figure 17.2 How gradients rephase.

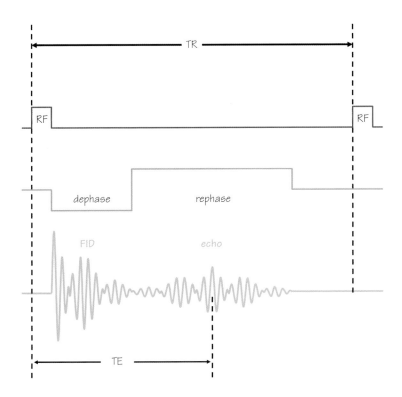

Figure 17.3 A basic gradient echo sequence showing how a bipolar application of the frequency-encoding gradient produces a gradient echo.

Gradient echo pulse sequences are sequences that use a gradient to rephase spins, as opposed to a 180° RF pulse used in spin echo sequences.

Mechanism

• The radio frequency excitation and relaxation pattern used in gradient echo consists of an RF excitation pulse followed by a relaxation period and a gradient reversal to produce rephasing of the spins. The magnitude and duration of the RF excitation pulse selected determines the **flip angle**, i.e. the angle through which the NMV moves away from B_0 during resonance (see Chapter 4).

• A transverse component of magnetization is created, the magnitude of which is less than in spin echo, where all the longitudinal magnetization is converted to transverse magnetization. When a flip angle other than 90° is used, only part of the longitudinal magnetization is converted to transverse magnetization, which precesses in the transverse plane and induces a signal in the receiver coil. Therefore the SNR in gradient echo sequences is less than in spin echo sequences (see Chapter 40) (Figure 17.1).

• After the RF pulse is withdrawn, the FID is immediately produced due to inhomogeneities in the magnetic field. Dephasing therefore occurs before T1 and T2 processes have had time to develop.

• The magnetic moments within the transverse component of magnetization dephase, and are then rephased by a **gradient**.

• A gradient causes a change in the magnetic field strength that changes the precessional frequency and phase of spins (see Chapter 56). This mechanism rephases the magnetic moments so that a signal is received by the receiver coil. This signal is called a **gradient echo** as gradient rather than an RF pulse was used to create it (Figure 17.2).

• Gradient rephasing is less efficient than RF rephasing. Gradient rephasing does not reverse nuclei that have been dephased from inhomogeneities in the main field. Gradient echo images therefore contain T2* effects such as increased noise and magnetic susceptibility artefact (see Chapter 47). Therefore T2 weighted gradient echo images are usually called T2* to reflect the presence of T2* effects. Gradient rephasing is faster than RF rephasing and therefore these sequences have shorter TEs and TRs than spin echo. As a result, scan times are short.

In a gradient echo pulse sequence, rephasing is performed by the **frequency encoding gradient** (see Chapter 30).

• The nuclei are dephased with a negative gradient pulse. The negative gradient slows down the slow nuclei even further, and speeds up the fast ones. This accelerates the dephasing process.

• The gradient polarity is then reversed to positive. The positive gradient speeds up the slow nuclei and slows down the fast ones. The nuclei rephase and produce a gradient echo (Figure 17.3).

• Gradient echo images are more sensitive to external magnetic field imperfections because T2* dephasing effects, produced by these inhomogeneities, are not eliminated by gradient rephasing.

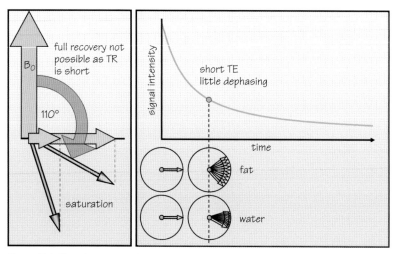

Figure 18.1 T1 weighting in gradient echo.

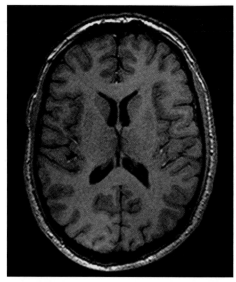

Figure 18.2 Axial T1 weighted gradient echo image of the brain.

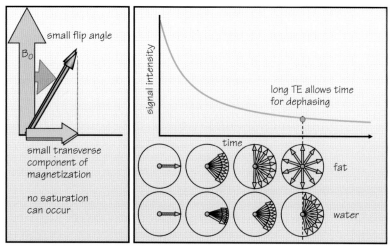

Figure 18.3 T2* weighting in gradient echo.

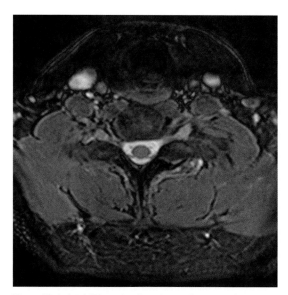

Figure 18.4 Axial T2* weighted gradient echo image of the cervical spine.

Contrast

As in spin echo imaging, the TR controls T1 weighting. The TR used in gradient echo is usually much shorter than in spin echo. This normally increases saturation and therefore T1 weighting, especially if the flip angle is large. To overcome this, the flip angle is reduced to less than 90° so that the NMV is predominantly in the longitudinal plane. This prevents saturation so the TR can be reduced.

• **In gradient echo sequences the TR and flip angle together, control T1/proton density weighting.**

The TE determines the amount of T2 dephasing that occurs before the NMV is rephased and therefore the amount of T2 relaxation affecting image contrast. The longer the TE, the more T2 contrast in the image. As gradient rephasing is less efficient than RF rephasing at removing inhomogeneity effects, they contain more residual T2* effects than spin echo. As a result the term **T2* weighting** is used in gradient echo imaging.

• **In gradient echo sequences the TE controls T2* weighting.**

Typical values

T1 weighting (Figures 18.1 and 18.2)

• Use a TR and flip angle to produce maximum T1 effects. The flip angle must shift the majority of the NMV towards the transverse plane to produce saturation. The **flip angle must be large**.

• The TR must not permit nuclei in the majority of tissues to recover to the longitudinal axis prior to the repetition of the next RF excitation pulse. Therefore the **TR must be short**.

• Use a TE to produce minimum T2* effects. The TE should limit the amount of dephasing that occurs before the echo is regenerated. Therefore the **TE must be short**.

For T1 weighting:

• **TR:** <50 ms (short)
• **Flip angle:** 60–120° (large)
• **TE:** <5 ms (short)

T2* weighting (Figures 18.3 and 18.4)

• The TE should permit maximum dephasing to occur before the signal is generated to produce maximum T2* effects. **The TE must be long.**

• The flip angle must shift only a minimum of the NMV towards the transverse plane. Small flip angles ensure that the majority of the net magnetization components remain in the longitudinal axis to prevent saturation. **The flip angle must be small.**

• **The TR must be long** enough to prevent saturation but can be reduced without producing significant saturation because of the small flip angle.

For T2* weighting:

• **TR:** >50 ms (long)
• **Flip angle:** <30° (small)
• **TE:** 15 ms (relatively long)

Proton density weighting

• Select TR and flip angle to produce minimum T1 effects and a TE to produce minimum T2* effects. As a result proton density predominates. The **flip angle must be small** so that the majority of the NMV remains in the longitudinal axis and therefore saturation and T1 weighting is minimized.

• **The TR must be long** to also minimize saturation and T1 effects.

• **The TE must be short** to minimize the T2* effects.

For proton density weighting:

• **TR:** >50 ms (long)
• **Flip angle:** 5–20° (small)
• **TE:** 5 ms (short)

Table 18.1 Parameters used in gradient echo

	TR	TE	Flip angle
T1 weighting	short	short	large
T2 weighting	long	long	small
PD weighting	long	short	small

19 The steady state

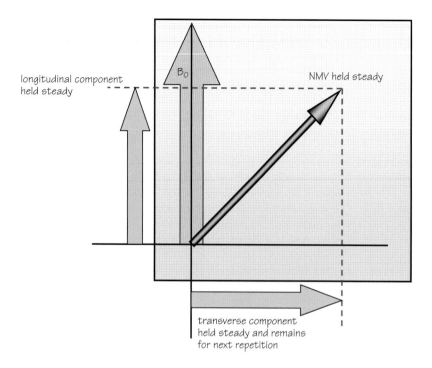

Figure 19.1 The steady state.

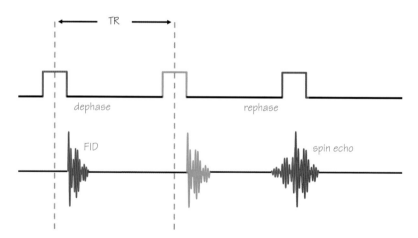

Figure 19.2 Echo formation part 1.

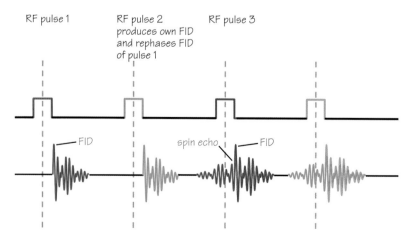

Figure 19.3 Echo formation part 2.

The **steady state** is defined as a stable condition that does not change over time. For this to occur any energy put into the system over time must equal any energy lost by the system in the same time period.

In MR, energy is put into the patient via the RF excitation pulse applied to a slice every TR. The quantity of energy applied during excitation is determined by the amplitude and duration of the RF pulse and results in a flip angle of a certain magnitude (see Chapter 4). The amount of energy lost is determined by the TR period as this is the time allowed for spin lattice energy transfer (see Chapter 6). To maintain the steady state, the TR and flip angle must be selected to ensure that the amount of energy given to the patient via excitation (as determined by the flip angle) more or less equals the amount of energy lost during relaxation (as determined by the TR).

• **To maintain the steady state the TR must be less than 50 ms and the flip angle between 30° and 45°.**

The steady state is maintained when the TR is shorter than both the T1 and T2 relaxation times of all the tissues. If the TR is longer than this, unachievably large flip angles would be required to maintain the steady state. Most gradient echo sequences utilize the steady state because the TRs are so short that the fastest scan times are permitted. However, when a very short TR is selected there is no time for the transverse magnetization to decay before the sequence is repeated again. The only process that has time to occur is T2*. Therefore the NMV does not really move between each TR and is held 'steady' (Figure 19.1). Because the transverse magnetization also does not have time to decay, its magnitude accumulates over successive TRs. This **residual transverse magnetization** affects image contrast as its presence is detected by the receiver coil. Tissues containing a high proportion of water, with long T2 decay times, appear bright as they remain in the transverse plane longer than tissues with short T2 decay times.

Echo generation in the steady state

As transverse magnetization does not have time to decay in the steady state, it builds up across successive TR periods and is rephased by each RF excitation pulse. Although the primary purpose of an excitation pulse is resonance, it will also rephase spins still present in the transverse plane and produce an echo if allowed to do so. This occurs because every RF pulse, regardless of its net magnitude, is able to rephase spins and produce an echo. Indeed all RF pulses, regardless of their net magnitude (as determined by the flip angle), are able to excite and rephase spins. In spin echo sequences this secondary effect is destroyed so that resonant (excitation) pulses only result in resonance, and rephasing pulses only result in rephasing spins to produce a spin echo. However, in the steady state these secondary effects are not eliminated and hence every RF excitation pulse applied both results in resonance (and therefore an FID when this pulse is removed) and also rephases any transverse magnetization to produce an echo. This occurs thus:

• Every TR, an excitation pulse is applied. When the RF pulse is switched off an FID is produced due to relaxation mechanisms (see Chapter 6).

• In the next TR period, another excitation pulse is applied which also produces its own FID. However, it also rephases spins still in the transverse plane from the previous RF pulse and a spin echo results.

• Each RF pulse therefore not only produces its own FID, but also rephases the residual transverse magnetization produced from previous excitations.

As the magnetic moments of nuclei take as long to rephase as they took to dephase, the echo from the first excitation pulse occurs at the same time as the third excitation pulse. This echo is called a **stimulated echo** (Figures 19.2 and 19.3). This process continues throughout the sequence. In gradient echo sequences that utilize the steady state there are therefore two signals available to produce the final gradient echo that is used to form the image:

• The **FID** which is produced as a result of inhomogeneities. This contains mainly T1 weighted information, especially if the TE is short.

• The **stimulated echo** which is the residual transverse magnetization, created across several TR periods, and contains mainly T2 weighted information, especially if the TE is long.

Most gradient echo sequences that use the steady state can be described according to which of these signals they use to generate an image and therefore explain the contrast they produce.

20 Coherent gradient echo

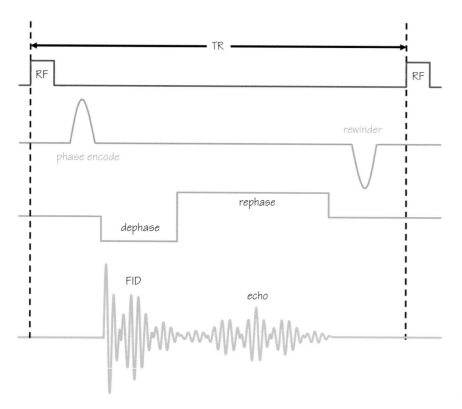

Figure 20.1 *Coherent gradient echo sequence.*

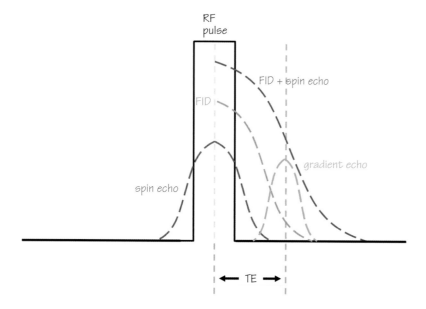

Figure 20.2 *Echo generation in coherent gradient echo.*

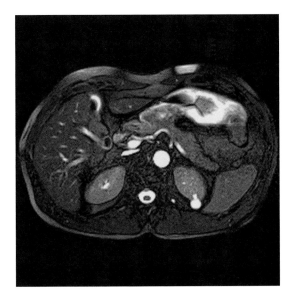

Figure 20.3 Axial coherent gradient echo image of the abdomen.

The main types of gradient echo sequence are:
- **coherent** or rewind sequences (Table 20.1);
- incoherent or spoiled sequences;
- steady-state free precession;
- balanced gradient echo.

Mechanism

This sequence uses:
- A gradient instead of a 180° rephasing pulse to rephase the echo.
- The steady state by using very short TRs and medium flip angles so that there is residual transverse magnetization 'left over' when the next excitation pulse is delivered. This residual magnetization is rephased by each excitation pulse to produce a stimulated echo (see Chapter 19).
- A **rewinder/rephasing gradient** to amplify the effect of both the FID and the stimulated echo by maintaining their coherency. This gradient is a reversal of the phase encoding gradient. This means that coherency is preserved. This process is called **rewinding** and both the FID and the stimulated echo are used to produce the gradient echo that forms the resultant image (Figures 20.1 and 20.2). Therefore images contain both T1 and T2* contrast but T2* effects dominate, especially if the TE is long. This is because the stimulated echo that is formed from the residual transverse magnetization is mainly made up of tissues containing a high proportion of water, with a long T2 decay time, because these tissues maintain their phase coherency longer than tissues with a short T2 decay time. These tissues (e.g. blood, CSF and synovial fluid) are therefore hyperintense on the image. These scans are often therefore said to produce an angiographic, myelographic or arthrographic appearance.

Typical values

As coherent gradient echo sequences utilize the steady state, the TR and the flip angle must be at values to achieve this. The TE determines how much T2* has occurred when the echo is regenerated. Coherent gradient echo sequences are primarily used to achieve T2* weighting using the following parameters:
- **TR short** (steady state): 35 ms
- **Flip angle medium** (steady state): 30°
- **TE long** (maximize T2*): 15 ms

Uses

This sequence should be used when T2* weighted images (bright blood, water or CSF) are required with good temporal resolution, for example:
- Breath-hold T2* imaging (Figure 20.3);
- Cine imaging of the heart;
- MR angiography (MRA);
- Volume imaging with T2* weighting.

Table 20.1 Coherent gradient echo acronyms

Philips	FFE
GE	GRASS
Siemens	FISP

21 Incoherent gradient echo

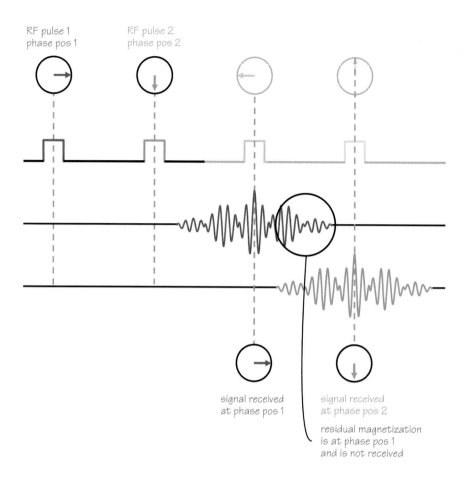

RF pulse 1
phase pos 1

RF pulse 2
phase pos 2

signal received
at phase pos 1

signal received
at phase pos 2

residual magnetization
is at phase pos 1
and is not received

Figure 21.1 Incoherent gradient echo sequence.

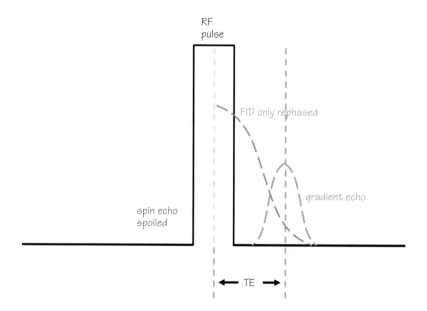

RF
pulse

FID only rephased

gradient echo

spin echo
spoiled

TE

Figure 21.2 Echo generation in incoherent gradient echo.

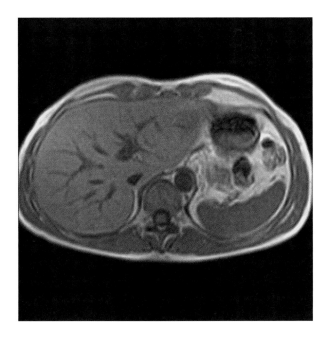

Figure 21.3 Axial incoherent gradient echo image of the abdomen.

The main types of gradient echo sequence are:
- coherent or rewind sequences;
- **incoherent** or spoiled sequences (Table 21.1);
- steady-state free precession;
- balanced gradient echo.

Mechanism

This sequence:
- Uses a gradient instead of a 180° rephasing pulse to rephase the echo.
- Utilizes the steady state by using very short TRs and medium flip angles so that there is residual transverse magnetization 'left over' when the next excitation pulse is delivered.
- Eliminates this magnetization so that tissues with long T2 times are not allowed to dominate image contrast but T1/proton density contrast prevails. This is achieved by **RF spoiling**.
- **RF spoiling** applies RF excitation pulses at different phases every TR so that the residual transverse magnetization has different phase values than the transverse magnetization most recently created (Figure 21.1).
- The residual transverse magnetization is therefore differentiated from that most recently created because it has a different phase value.
- The residual transverse magnetization and therefore the stimulated echo are not sampled. Only the FID is used to produce the gradient echo that forms the resultant image. Therefore images contain mainly T1 contrast (Figure 21.2).

Typical values

The incoherent gradient echo sequence utilizes the steady state, so the TR and the flip angle must be at values to achieve this. The TE is as a short as possible to minimize T2* effects. Incoherent gradient echo is primarily used for T1 weighting with the following parameters:
- **TR short** (steady state): 35 ms
- **Flip angle medium** (steady state): 35°
- **TE short** (minimize T2*): 5 ms

Uses

This sequence should be used when T1 weighted images are required with good temporal resolution:
- 3D volume acquisitions acquire data from a volume of tissue. A whole slab is excited (but not slice selected) and during the encoding process the slab is phase shifted into slices (**slice encoding**). As slice encoding is another form of phase encoding, the number of slices increases the scan time proportionally (see Chapter 37). 3D volume acquisitions are therefore quite lengthy scans and are often used with fast sequences. Volume acquisition allows very thin slices to be obtained at many slice locations. The data acquired can then be used to view the slab in any plane.
- 2D breath-hold T1 weighted sequences (Figure 21.3).
- Dynamic contrast enhanced images.

Table 21.1 Incoherent gradient echo acronyms

Philips	T1 FFE
GE	SPGR
Siemens	FLASH

22 Steady-state free precession

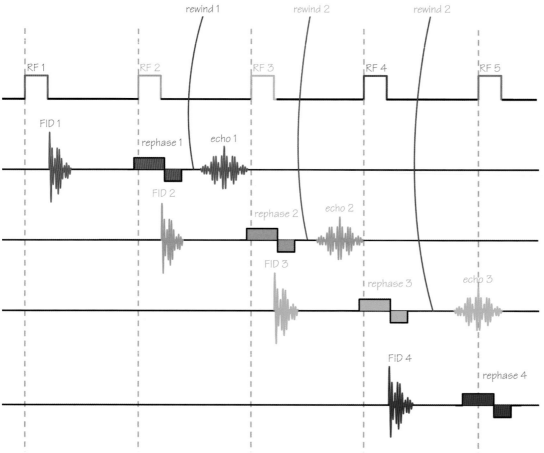

Figure 22.1 SSFP sequence.

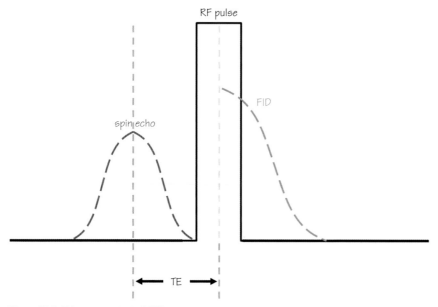

Figure 22.2 Echo generation in SSFP.

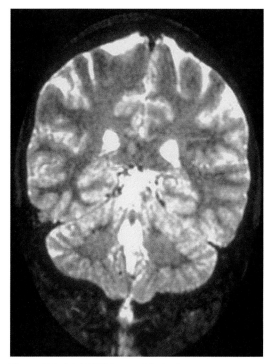

Figure 22.3 Axial SSFP image of the brain.

Table 22.1 Steady-state free precession acronyms

Philips	T2 FFE
GE	SSFP
Siemens	PSIF

The main types of gradient echo sequence are:
• coherent or rewind sequences;
• incoherent or spoiled sequences;
• **steady-state free precession** or **SSFP** (Table 22.1);
• balanced gradient echo.

Gradient echo sequences do not demonstrate true T2 weighting because the TE is never long enough to measure a tissues T2 decay time. A TE of at least 70 ms is required to demonstrate true T2 weighting, and in gradient echo sequences the TE is rarely higher than 15 ms. SSFP is a steady state sequence that obtains images that have a sufficiently long TE to measure T2 decay when using the steady state while still using a short TR. This is achieved in the following manner.

Mechanism
• In SSFP, the steady state is maintained by using a flip angle between 30° and 45° in conjunction with a TR of less than 50 ms.

• Every TR an excitation pulse is applied. When the RF is switched off a FID is produced.
• After the first TR period, another excitation pulse is applied which also produces its own FID. However, it also rephases the residual transverse magnetization still present from the previous excitation and produces a stimulated echo (see Chapter 19).
• As nuclei take as long to rephase after a 180° rephasing pulse as they took to dephase before it, the stimulated echo occurs at the same time as the third excitation pulse.
• In SSFP this stimulated echo must be sampled on its own. However in order to do this it must be moved away from the excitation pulse as RF cannot be transmitted and received at the same time.
• To achieve this, a rewinder gradient is used to speed up the rephasing process after the RF rephasing has begun. Rewinding moves the echo so that it occurs sooner than usual and it no longer occurs at the same time as an excitation pulse. In this way, the stimulated echo can be received and data from it, collected. This data is used to form the image (Figures 22.1 and 22.2).

The resultant echo demonstrates more true T2 weighting than conventional gradient echo sequences. This is because the TE is now longer than the TR. In SSFP, there are usually two TEs:
• the **actual TE** (time between the stimulated echo and the next excitation pulse);
• the **effective TE** (time from the stimulated echo to the excitation pulse that created it. This is the TE that determines the T2 weighting of the image). Therefore:

the effective TE = (2 × TR) minus actual TE

This means that the effective TE is longer than the TR and can be long enough to measure true T2. From the equation above it can be seen that the shorter the actual TE, the higher the effective TE and hence increased T2 weighting.

Typical values
• **Flip angle:** 30–45°
• **TR:** <50 ms
• **TE (actual):** 7 ms

Uses
SSFP sequences are used to rapidly acquire images that demonstrate true T2 weighting (Figure 22.3). With the advent of turbo spin echo, however, this sequence is not usually used for this purpose. But the principle of echo shifting (moving an echo to increase the effective TE) in conjunction with short TRs is used in many techniques including perfusion imaging (see Chapter 25).

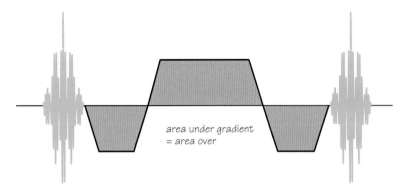

area under gradient
= area over

Figure 23.1 Balanced gradient scheme in balanced gradient echo.

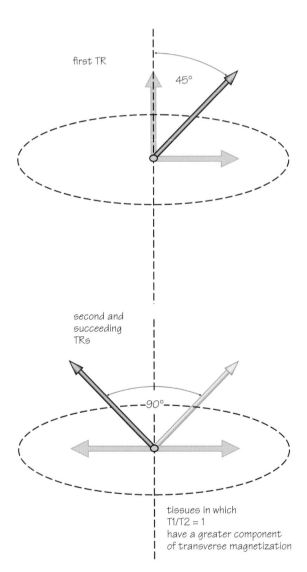

first TR

45°

second and
succeeding
TRs

90°

tissues in which
T1/T2 = 1
have a greater component
of transverse magnetization

Figure 23.2 Alternating RF pulses balanced gradient echo.

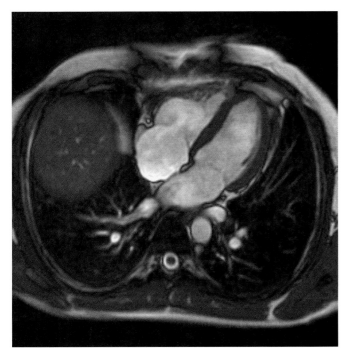

Figure 23.3 Axial balanced gradient echo of the heart.

Table 23.1 Balanced gradient echo acronyms

Philips	BFFE
GE	FIESTA
Siemens	True FISP

The main types of gradient echo sequence are called:
- coherent or rewind sequences;
- incoherent or spoiled sequences;
- steady state free precession;
- **balanced gradient echo** (Table 23.1).
  This sequence was developed to:
- reduce flow artefacts from high signal intensity areas;
- increase SNR and CNR in gradient echo sequences.

To reduce flow artefacts it is important to reduce the TR to a minimum so that there is less time for spins to exit the slice (see Chapter 50). SNR may be increased by increasing the flip angle (see Chapter 40). However, combining a very short TR with a large flip angle results in saturation and therefore an increase in T1 weighting. The purpose of balanced gradient echo is to use a large flip angle (that increases SNR) with a very short TR (that reduces flow artefacts) while at the same time reducing saturation and increasing T2* weighting. This is achieved in the following manner.

Mechanism

- A flow-compensated balanced gradient system is used to maintain coherency in flowing spins, thereby increasing their signal intensity (Figure 23.1) (see Chapter 50).
- A large flip angle (e.g. 90°) is selected but in the first TR only half this flip angle is applied (e.g. 45°). The RF excitation pulse creates transverse magnetization at a particular phase position in the transverse plane.
- In the second TR period a second excitation pulse is applied that creates transverse magnetization 180° out of phase with transverse magnetization created in the first TR period. This is achieved by applying the second RF pulse at a flip angle of −90° to the first excitation pulse.
- Saturation does not occur because the transverse magnetization created in the second TR period does not add to that created in the first TR period, since it has a different phase position on the transverse plane.
- This pattern is repeated throughout the sequence. Every TR the phase of the transverse magnetization is changed by alternating the flip angle between +90° and −90°, therefore creating transverse magnetization at a different phase each time. Saturation is therefore prevented despite using large flip angles and very short TRs, and T2* weighting can predominate.
- Large flip angles maximize SNR.
- Very short TRs minimize flow artefacts as there is less time for spins to exit the slice (Figure 23.2).

Typical values

- **Flip angle:** 90°
- **TE:** 10 ms
- **TR:** <10 ms

Uses

Although this sequence was primarily developed for use in cardiac imaging, it is also important whenever T2* weighted images are required in areas where flow causes motion artefact. Commonly this sequence is used in the central nervous system to reduce flow from CSF, e.g. the internal auditory meatus (IAM) and the cervical spine. However it is also used in the abdominal system to reduce flow artefacts in the biliary and circulatory systems (Figure 23.3). As the TR is so short, this sequence provides excellent temporal resolution and is also useful in volume imaging.

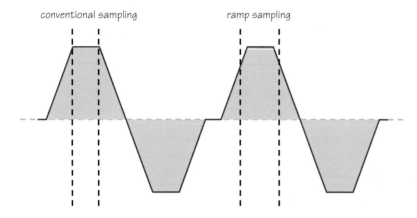

Figure 24.1 Conventional versus ramped sampling.

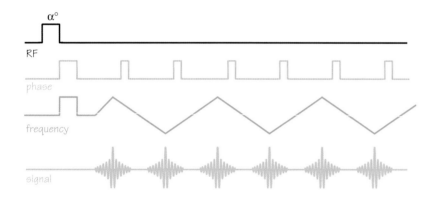

Figure 24.2 GE EPI sequence.

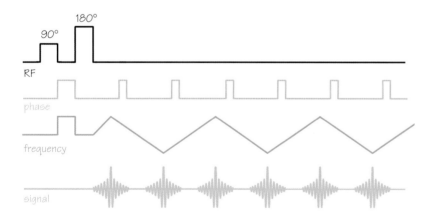

Figure 24.3 SE EPI sequence.

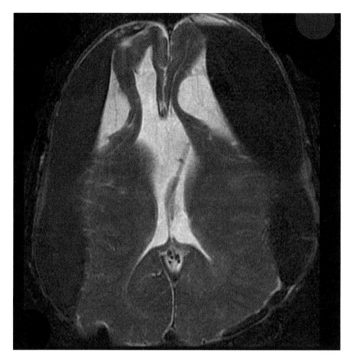

Figure 24.4 Axial SE EPI of the brain showing haemorrhage.

Very fast pulse sequences include faster versions of coherent and in-coherent gradient echo sequences or combinations of both (**hybrids**). Faster scan times are achieved in the following ways:
• applying only a portion of the RF excitation pulse, so that it takes much less time to apply and switch off;
• only a proportion of the echo is read (**partial echo**);
• using asymmetric gradients, which are faster to apply than conventional balanced gradients;
• sampling frequencies while the frequency-encoding gradient is still rising (**ramped sampling**) (Figure 24.1);
• filling K space in a single shot or in segments (see Chapter 39).

These measures ensure that the TE and TR are very short. TEs as low as 1 ms and TRs as low as 5 ms can be achieved in this manner enabling a 3D slab to be imaged in a single breath-hold. In addition, many ultra-fast sequences use extra pulses applied before the pulse sequence begins to premagnetize the tissue. In this way a certain contrast can be obtained. Premagnetization is usually achieved in two ways:
• a 180° pulse is applied before the pulse sequence begins. This inverts the NMV into full saturation and, at a specified delay time, the pulse sequence itself begins. This can be used to null signal from certain organs and tissues and is similar to inversion recovery. It is sometimes known as a **magnetization prepared** sequence.
• A 90°/180°/90° combination is applied before the pulse sequence begins. The first 90° pulse produces transverse magnetization. The 180° pulse rephases this, and at a specified time later the second 90° pulse is applied. This drives the any coherent transverse magnetization into the longitudinal plane, so that it is available to be flipped into the longitudinal plane when the pulse sequence begins again. This is used to produce T2 contrast and is sometimes known as **driven equilibrium**.

Weighting is achieved in these sequences by applying all the shallowest phase-encoding gradients first, and leaving the steep ones until the end of the pulse sequence. In this way, the effect of the premagnetization prevails as, when it is dominant, the central phase encodings (that produce the greatest signal amplitudes and determine the weighting of the sequence) are performed (see Chapter 39). By the end of the sequence, the premagnetization has decayed and this is when the low signal amplitudes are acquired.

Echo planar imaging

Echo planar imaging or **EPI** is an MR acquisition method that either fills all the lines of K space in a single repetition (single shot – SS) or in multiple sections (multishot – MS). In order to achieve this, multiple echoes are generated and each is phase encoded by a different slope of gradient to fill all the required lines of K space. Echoes are generated by oscillation of the frequency-encoding gradient and therefore K space is filled with data acquired from multiple gradient echoes. In order to fill all of K space in this way, the readout and phase-encoding gradients must rapidly switch on and off (see Chapter 38). This technique is called **SS-EPI** or **MS-EPI** depending on whether K space is filled in one repetition or several. There are many types of EPI sequence:
• **GE-EPI** uses a variable flip angle followed by EPI readout in K space (Figure 24.2);
• **SE-EPI** uses a 90°/180° followed by EPI readout in K space (Figures 24.3 and 24.4);
• **IR-EPI** uses a 180°/90°/180° followed by EPI readout in K space.
Note: Single or multishot techniques in which spin echoes are generated by 180° rephasing pulses instead of gradient echoes are called **single or multi-shot turbo spin echo** (**SS-TSE** or **MS-TSE**).

Gradient rephasing as used by SS-EPI or MS-EPI techniques is much faster than RF rephasing (as used by SS-TSE or MS-TSE) and involves no RF deposition to the patient but does require high-speed gradients. However, as inhomogeneity effects are not compensated for by gradient rephasing, artefacts are more abundant. EPI sequences place exceptional strains on the gradients and therefore gradient modifications are required.

Typical values

Either proton density or T2 weighting is achieved by selecting either a short or long effective TE which corresponds to the time interval between the excitation pulse and when the centre of K space is filled. In single-shot techniques, as there is only one excitation pulse, there is no repetition and as a result the TR is said to equal infinity, i.e. it is infinitely long. T1 weighting is only possible by applying an inverting pulse prior to the excitation pulse to produce saturation.

Uses

• Diffusion weighted imaging (see Chapter 25).
• Perfusion imaging (see Chapter 25).
• Functional imaging (see Chapter 26).
• Real-time cardiac imaging.
• Interventional techniques.
• Breath-hold techniques.

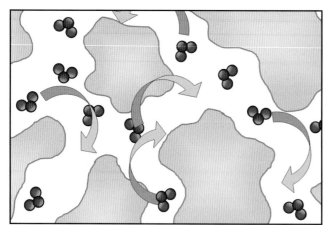

freely diffusing water

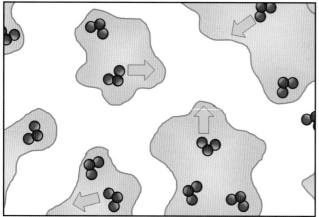

restricted water

Figure 25.1 Free and restricted diffusion.

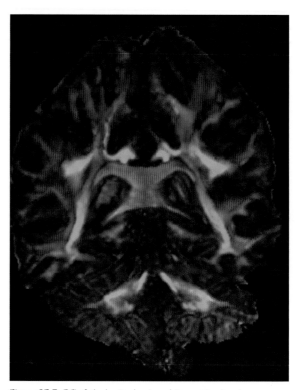

Figure 25.3 DTI of the brain showing white matter tracts.

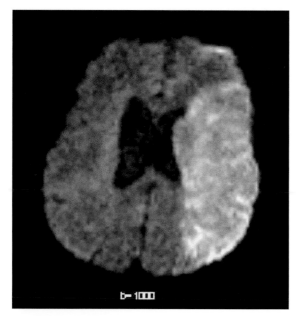

b = 1000

Figure 25.2 Axial DWI of the brain showing a left-sided infarct.

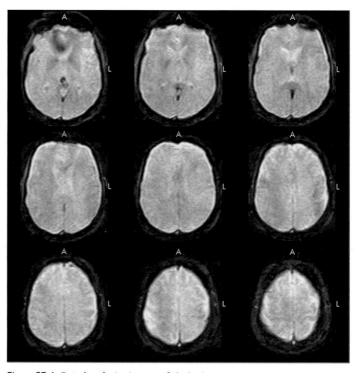

Figure 25.4 Set of perfusion images of the brain.

Diffusion weighted imaging

Diffusion is a term used to describe moving molecules due to random thermal motion. This motion is restricted by boundaries such as ligaments, membranes and macro-molecules and by pathology. The parameter used to describe the rate of diffusion in tissues is the **apparent diffusion coefficient** or **ADC**. Tissues in which diffusion is free have a high ADC whereas those with restricted diffusion have a low ADC (Figure 25.1).

Diffusion weighted images (DWI) are acquired by sensitizing this motion with the use of strong gradients. The gradient pulses are designed to cancel each other out if spins do not move, while moving spins experience phase shift. Signal attenuation therefore occurs in normal tissues with free random motion (high ADC) and high signal appears in tissues with restricted diffusion (low ADC). The amount of attenuation depends on the amplitude and the direction of the applied diffusion gradients and the ADC of the tissue. Diffusion gradients applied in the X, Y and Z axes (see Chapter 27) are combined to produce a diffusion weighted image (isotropic image). When the diffusion gradients are applied in only one direction, signal changes reflect direction of axons (anisotropic image).

Diffusion gradients must be strong to achieve enough diffusion weighting. Diffusion sensitivity is controlled by a parameter **'b'** that determines the diffusion attenuation by modification of the duration and amplitude of the diffusion gradient. 'b' is expressed in units of s/mm^2. Typical 'b' values range from 500 s/mm^2 to 1000 s/mm^2. As 'b' increases, diffusion weighting also increases and vice versa. The 'b' value is an extrinsic contrast parameter that controls how contrast is derived in a diffusion weighted image in that high 'b' values exaggerate the differences in a tissue's ADC values (an intrinsic contrast parameter) (see Chapter 5).

Clinical applications

DWI is commonly used in the diagnosis of stroke where areas of decreased diffusion, which represent infarction, are bright (Figure 25.2).

In early stroke, cells swell and absorb water from the extracellular space and diffusion is restricted. These changes are seen very shortly after the stroke and are helpful to visualize the locality and extent of an infarct before other modalities are able to visualize them. DWI is also useful in other areas such as the liver, prostate and breast to differentiate between malignant and benign lesions and to differentiate solid from cystic areas. Very strong multidirectional gradients may be used to map white matter tracts which have a lower ADC than surrounding grey matter. This technique is called **diffusion tensor imaging** or **DTI** (Figure 25.3). Other structures which contain fibres, such as muscle, may also be seen with this technique. Examples include skeletal muscle and the left ventricle.

Perfusion imaging

Perfusion is a measure of the quality of vascular supply to a tissue. Since vascular supply and metabolism are usually related, perfusion can also be used to measure tissue activity. **Perfusion imaging** utilizes a bolus injection of gadolinium administered intravenously during ultrafast T2* acquisitions. The contrast agent causes transient decreases in T2* in and around the micro-vasculature perfused with contrast. After data acquisition, a signal decay curve can be used to ascertain blood volume, transit time and measurement of perfusion. This curve is known as a **time intensity curve**. Time intensity curves for multiple images acquired during and after injection are combined to generate a **cerebral blood volume (CBV) map**. **Mean transit times (MTT)** of contrast through an organ or tissue can also be calculated.

Clinical applications

Perfusion imaging is commonly used in evaluation of ischaemic disease or metabolism. On the CBV map, areas of low perfusion (e.g. stroke) appear dark whereas areas of higher perfusion (e.g. malignancy) appear bright (Figure 25.4).

Functional imaging techniques

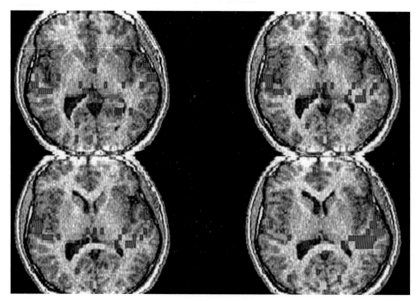

Figure 26.1 BOLD images of the brain. Functional areas in red.

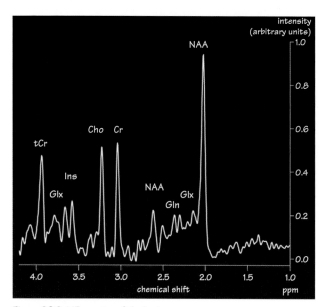

Figure 26.2 MR spectra of the brain.

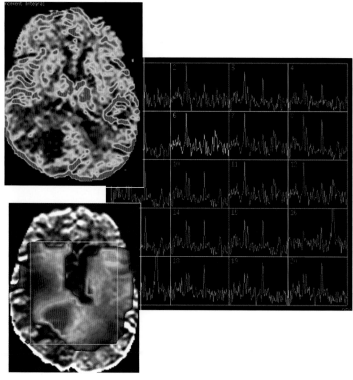

Figure 26.3 Multi voxel MRS technique.

Functional MR imaging (fMRI) is a rapid MR imaging technique that acquires images of the brain during activity or stimulus and at rest. The two sets of images are then subtracted, demonstrating functional brain activity as the result of increased blood flow to the activated cortex.

BOLD imaging

The most important physiological effect that produces MR signal intensity changes between stimulus and rest is called **blood oxygenation level dependent** or **BOLD**. BOLD exploits differences in the magnetic susceptibility of oxyhaemoglobin and deoxyhaemoglobin.

• **Haemoglobin** is a molecule that contains iron and transports oxygen in the vascular system as oxygen binds directly to iron.

• **Oxyhaemoglobin** is a diamagnetic molecule in which the magnetic properties of iron are largely suppressed.

• **Deoxyhaemoglobin** is a paramagnetic molecule that creates an inhomogeneous magnetic field in its immediate vicinity that increases $T2^*$.

At rest, tissues use a substantial fraction of the blood flowing through the capillaries so venous blood contains an almost equal mix of oxyhaemoglobin and deoxyhaemoglobin. During exercise, however, when metabolism is increased, more oxygen is needed and hence more is extracted from the capillaries. The brain is very sensitive to low concentrations of oxyhaemoglobin and therefore the cerebral vascular system increases blood flow to the activated area. This causes a drop in deoxyhaemoglobin that results in a decrease in dephasing and a corresponding increase in signal intensity. Blood oxygenation increases during brain activity, and specific locations of the cerebral cortex are activated during specific tasks. For example, seeing activates the visual cortex, hearing the auditory cortex, finger tapping the motor cortex (Figure 26.1). More sophisticated tasks, including maze paradigms and other thought-provoking tasks, stimulate other brain cortices.

BOLD effects are very short lived and therefore require extremely rapid sequences such as EPI or fast gradient echo. The images are usually acquired with long TEs (40–70 ms) using echo-shifting techniques (see Chapter 22) while the task is modulated on and off. The 'off' images are then subtracted from the 'on' images and a more sophisticated statistical analysis is performed. Regions that were activated above some threshold level are overlaid onto anatomic images.

Clinical applications

The clinical applications are primarily in development of the understanding of brain function including evaluation of stroke, epilepsy, pain and behavioural problems.

Spectroscopy

Spectroscopy provides a frequency spectrum of a given tissue based on the molecular and chemical structures of that tissue (Figure 26.2). Peak size and placement within the measured spectrum provide information on how an atom is bonded to a molecule. Most clinical spectroscopy looks at hydrogen but advanced forms are able to evaluate other MR active nuclei. Spatial localization can be achieved by using the **stimulated-echo acquisition mode** or **STEAM**. The localized volume is generated via stimulated echoes from spins excited by three 90° RF pulses, and the conventional STEAM sequence detects the stimulated echo. A slice selective RF pulse is applied in conjunction with an X magnetic field gradient. This excites spins in an YZ plane. A 180° slice selective RF pulse is applied in conjunction with a Y magnetic field gradient. This rotates spins located in an XZ plane. A second 180° slice selective RF pulse is applied in conjunction with a Z magnetic field gradient. The second 180° pulse excites spins in a XY plane. The second echo is recorded as the signal. This echo represents the signal from those spins in the intersection of the three planes. Fourier transformation of the echo produces a spectrum of the spins located at the intersection of the three planes.

Clinical applications

Spectroscopy is now becoming a routine part of clinical imaging to evaluate tissue metabolism and identification of tumour types (Figure 26.3).

27 Gradient functions

main magnet windings
gradient coil
subtracts from B_0
adds to B_0
+ + + + + + + +
−
+
−

Figure 27.1 A gradient coil.

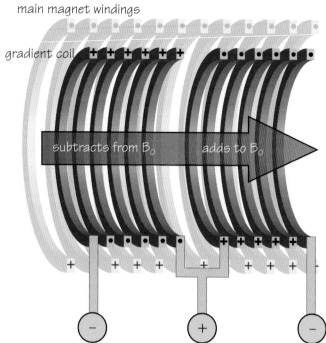

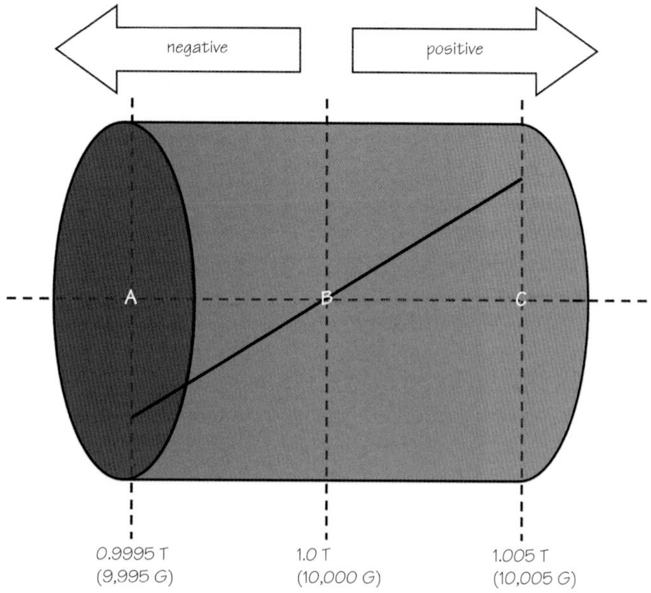

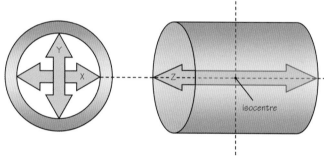

negative
positive
A
B
C
0.9995 T
(9,995 G)
1.0 T
(10,000 G)
1.005 T
(10,005 G)

Figure 27.2 Gradients and changing field strength.

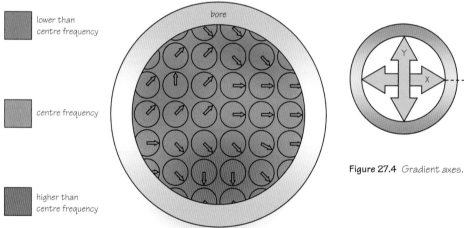

lower than
centre frequency
centre frequency
higher than
centre frequency
bore

Figure 27.3 How gradients change frequency and phase.

Y
X
Z
isocentre

Figure 27.4 Gradient axes.

Gradients are coils of wire that, when a current is passed through them, alter the magnetic field strength of the magnet in a controlled and predictable way. They add or subtract from the existing field in a linear fashion so that the magnetic field strength at any point along the gradient is known (Figure 27.1). When a gradient is applied the following occur:

• At **isocentre** the field strength remains unchanged even when the gradient is switched on.

• At a certain distance away from isocentre the field strength either increases or decreases. The magnitude of the change depends on the distance from isocentre and the strength of the gradient (Figure 27.2).

• The slope of the gradient signifies the rate of change of the magnetic field strength along its length. The **strength** or **amplitude** of the gradient is determined by **how much current** is applied to the gradient coil. Larger currents create steeper gradients so that the change in field strength over distance is greater. The reverse is true of smaller currents.

• The **polarity** of the gradient determines which end of the gradient produces a higher field strength than isocentre (positive) and which a lower field strength than isocentre (negative). The polarity of the gradient is determined by the **direction of the current** flowing through the coil. As coils are circular, current either flows clockwise or anticlockwise.

• The **maximum amplitude** of the gradient determines the maximum achievable **resolution**.

• The speed with which gradients can be switched on and off are called the **rise time** and **slew rate**. Both of these factors determine the maximum scan speeds of a system (see Chapter 56).

How gradients work

The precessional frequency of the magnetic moments of nuclei is proportional to the magnetic field strength experienced by them (as stated by the Larmor equation; see Chapter 3). The frequency of signal received from the patient can be changed according to its position along the gradient. The precessional phase is also affected as faster magnetic moments gain phase compared with their slower neighbours.

Imposing a gradient magnetic field therefore:

• Changes the field strength in a linear fashion across a distance in the patient.

• Changes the precessional **frequency** of magnetic moments of nuclei in a linear fashion across a distance in the patient.

• Changes the precessional **phase** of magnetic moments of nuclei in a linear fashion across a distance in the patient (Figure 27.3).

These characteristics can be used to **encode** the MR signal in three dimensions. In order to do this there must be three orthogonal sets of gradients situated within the bore of the magnet. They are named according to the axis along which they work.

The **Z gradient** alters the magnetic field strength along the **Z axis**.

The **Y gradient** alters the magnetic field strength along the **Y axis**.

The **X gradient** alters the magnetic field strength along the **X axis**.

The **isocentre** is the centre of all three gradients. The field strength here does not change even when a gradient is applied (Figure 27.4).

There are only three gradients but they are used to perform many important functions during a pulse sequence. One of these functions is **spatial encoding**, i.e. spatially locating a signal in three dimensions. In order to do this, three separate functions are necessary. Usually each gradient performs one of the following tasks. The gradient used for each task depends on the plane of the scan and on which gradient the operator selects to perform frequency or phase encoding.

(1) **Slice selection** – locating a slice in the scan plane selected.

(2) Spatially locating signal along the short axis of the image. This is called **phase encoding**.

(3) Spatially locating signal along the long axis of the image. This is called **frequency encoding** (Table 27.1).

Table 27.1 Gradient axes in orthogonal imaging

	Slice selection	Phase encoding	Frequency encoding
Sagittal	X	Y	Z
Axial (body)	Z	Y	X
Axial (head)	Z	X	Y
Coronal	Y	X	Z

28 Slice selection

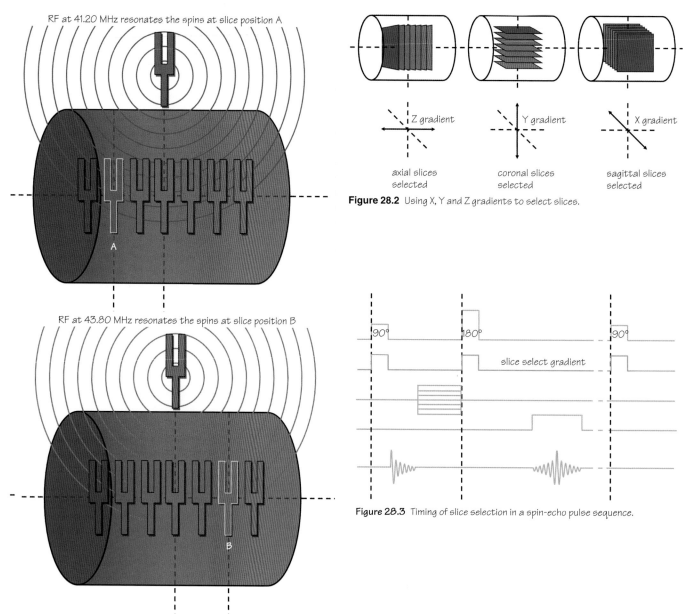

RF at 41.20 MHz resonates the spins at slice position A

A

RF at 43.80 MHz resonates the spins at slice position B

B

Figure 28.1 Slice selection.

Z gradient

axial slices
selected

Y gradient

coronal slices
selected

X gradient

sagittal slices
selected

Figure 28.2 Using X, Y and Z gradients to select slices.

90°   180°   90°

slice select gradient

Figure 28.3 Timing of slice selection in a spin-echo pulse sequence.

Mechanism

As a gradient alters the magnetic field strength of the magnet linearly, the magnetic moments of nuclei within a specific slice location along the gradient have a unique precessional frequency when the gradient is on. A slice can therefore be selectively excited by transmitting RF at that unique precessional frequency.

Example: a 1T field strength magnet with a gradient imposed that has changed the field strength between slice A and B causing a change in precessional frequency between slice A and B of 2.6 MHz (Figure 28.1).

- The precessional frequency of magnetic moments between slice A and B has changed by 2.6 MHz.
- To excite nuclei in slice A an RF pulse of 41.20 MHz must be applied.
- Slice B and all other slices are not excited because their precessional frequencies are different due to the influence of the gradient.
- To excite slice B, another RF pulse with a frequency of 43.80 MHz must be applied. Nuclei in slice A do not resonate after the application of this pulse because they are spinning at a different frequency.

The scan plane selected determines which gradient performs slice selection. In a superconducting system (in an open magnet system, the Z and Y axes are transposed):

- The **Z** gradient selects **axial** slices, so that nuclei in the patient's head spin at a different frequency to those in the feet.
- The **Y** gradient selects **coronal** slices, so that nuclei at the back of the patient spin at a different frequency to those at the front.
- The **X** gradient selects **sagittal** slices, so that nuclei on the right-hand side of the patient spin at a different frequency to those on the left (Figure 28.2).
- A combination of any two gradients selects **oblique** slices.

Slice thickness

In order to attain slice thickness, a range of frequencies must be transmitted to produce resonance across the whole slice (and therefore to excite the whole slice). This range of frequencies is called a **bandwidth** and because RF is being transmitted at this instant, it is specifically called the **transmit bandwidth**.

- The slice thickness is determined by the slope of the slice select gradient and the transmit bandwidth. It affects inplane spatial resolution (see Chapter 42).
- **Thin** slices require a **steep** slope and **narrow** transmit bandwidth, and improve spatial resolution.
- **Thick** slices require a **shallow** slope and **broad** transmit bandwidth, and decrease spatial resolution.

A slice is therefore excited by transmitting RF with a centre frequency corresponding to the middle of the slice, and a bandwidth and gradient slope according to the thickness of the slice required. The **slice gap** or **skip** is the space between slices. Too small a gap in relation to the slice thickness can lead to an artefact called **cross-excitation**.

The slice select gradient is switched on during the delivery of the RF excitation pulse. It is switched on in the positive direction. The slice select gradient is also switched on during the 180° pulse in spin echo sequences so that the RF rephasing pulse can be delivered specifically to the selected slice (Figure 28.3).

29 Phase encoding

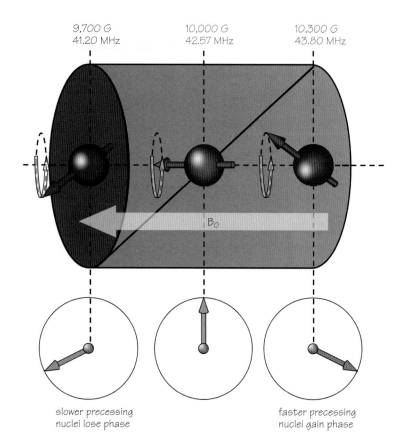

9,700 G
41.20 MHz

10,000 G
42.57 MHz

10,300 G
43.80 MHz

B₀

slower precessing
nuclei lose phase

faster precessing
nuclei gain phase

Figure 29.1 Phase encoding.

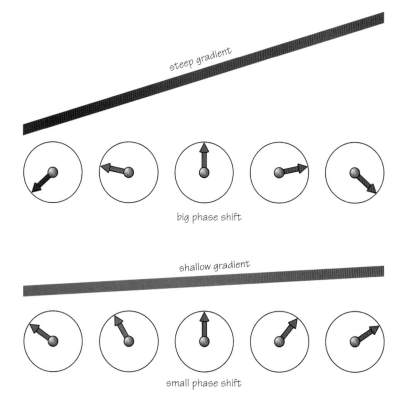

steep gradient

big phase shift

shallow gradient

small phase shift

Figure 29.2 Steep and shallow phase encodings.

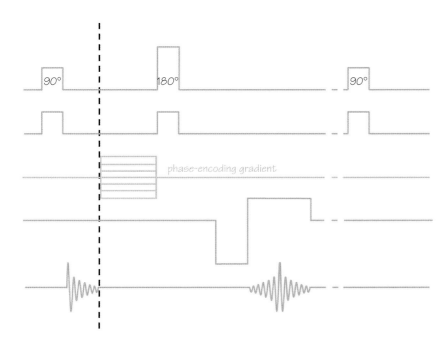

Figure 29.3 Timing of phase encoding in a spin-echo pulse sequence.

After a slice has been select and the slice select gradient switched off, the magnetic field strength experienced by nuclei within the excited slice equals the field strength of the system. The precessional frequency of spins within the slice is therefore equal to the Larmor frequency. The frequency of the signal from the slice also equals the Larmor frequency, regardless of the location of each signal within the slice. The system therefore has to use gradients to gain two-dimensional information representing the spatial location of the spins within the slice. When a gradient is switched on, the precessional frequency of a spin is determined by its physical location on the gradient.

Mechanism

The gradient changes the **phase** of the magnetic moment of each nucleus or spin. The phase of a magnetic moment is its place on the circular precessional path at any moment in time (see Chapter 3). It can be compared with the position of the minute hand on a clock.

• A nucleus that experiences a higher magnetic field strength when the gradient is switched on, gains phase relative to its position without the gradient on. This is because when a spin precesses at a higher frequency it is travelling faster and therefore moves further around 'the clock' than it would have done with the gradient off.

• If a nucleus experiences a lower magnetic field strength with the gradient on, its magnetic moment slows down relative to its speed or frequency with the gradient off, and loses phase.

• Therefore, the presence of a gradient along one axis of the image causes a **phase shift** of nuclei along the length of the gradient (Figure 29.1). The degree of phase shift relative to isocentre depends on its distance from isocentre and the slope of the phase gradient.

• When the phase-encoding gradient is switched off, nuclei return to the Larmor frequency but their phase shift remains, i.e. they all travel at the same speed around the clock but their positions on the clock are different. This phase shift is used to spatially locate the nuclei (and therefore signal) along one dimension of the image.

• The **slope** or amplitude of the phase-encoding gradient determines the degree of phase shift. Steeper gradients produce a greater phase shift between two points than shallower gradients (Figure 29.2). Steeper gradients increase the **phase matrix** (see Chapter 42) and therefore the resolution of the image along the phase axis.

The phase-encoding gradient is switched on after the RF excitation pulse has been switched off, and the amplitude and polarity of the gradient is altered for each phase-encoding step in standard sequences (see Chapter 32) (Figure 29.3).

30 Frequency encoding

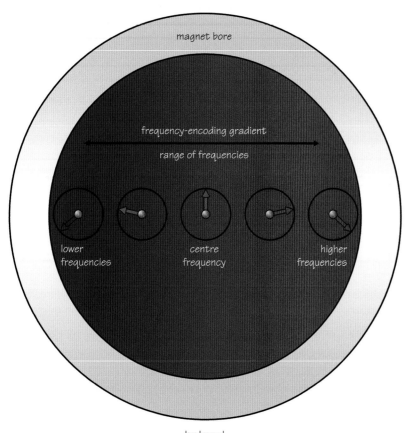

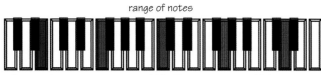

Figure 30.1 Frequency encoding.

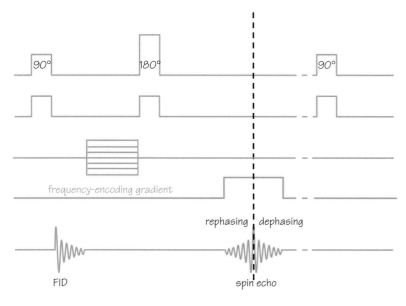

Figure 30.2 Timing of frequency encoding in a spin echo pulse sequence.

After a slice has been selected and the slice select gradient switched off, the magnetic field strength experienced by nuclei within the excited slice equals the field strength of the system. The precessional frequency of spins within the slice is equal to the Larmor frequency. The frequency of the signal from the slice also equals the Larmor frequency, regardless of the location of each signal within the slice. The system has to use gradients to gain two-dimensional information representing the spatial location of the spins within the slice. When a gradient is switched on, the precessional frequency of a nucleus is determined by its physical location on the gradient. The change in frequency that this gradient produces is similar to the range of notes on a keyboard.

Mechanism

A gradient corresponding to the long axis dimension of anatomy in the image is switched on to locate signal along this axis. The frequency change caused by the gradient is used to locate each signal. It produces a **frequency change** or **frequency shift** in the following manner:
- The spins of nuclei experiencing a higher magnetic field strength due to the gradient speed up; i.e. their precessional frequencies increase (similar to a high note on a keyboard).
- The spins of nuclei experiencing a lower magnetic field strength due to the presence of the gradient slow down; i.e. their precessional frequencies decrease (similar to a low note on a keyboard) (Figure 30.1).

- This is called **frequency encoding** and results in a **frequency shift** of nuclei relative to their position on the gradient.
- The **frequency-encoding gradient** is switched on during the echo. It is often called the **readout** gradient because, during its application, frequencies within the signal are read by the system. The echo is usually centred to the middle of the gradient application and the readout gradient is usually switched on in the positive direction (see Chapter 32) (Figure 30.2).
- The **slope** of the frequency-encoding gradient determines the **size of the FOV** in the frequency direction and therefore image resolution (see Chapter 42).

Learning point

Each system has a minimum length of time required to switch all three gradients on and off. The speed with which it can do this depends on the sophistication of the gradients, their amplifiers and switching mechanisms. Steep gradients take longer to apply than shallow ones and an echo cannot be received until each gradient function has been performed. The selection of thin slices, high phase matrices or a small FOV require each gradient to have a steep gradient slope. This results in the minimum TE increasing so that each of these gradients can be applied before the echo is read.

31 K space – what is it?

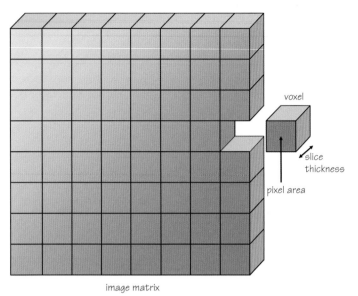

Figure 31.1 The voxel.

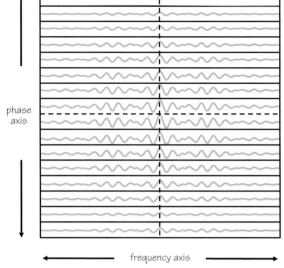

Figure 31.3 K space axes.

Figure 31.2 Fast Fourier transform.

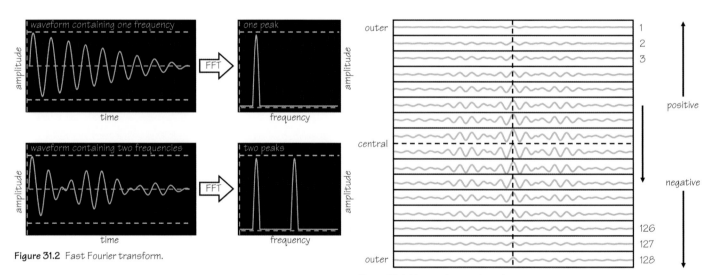

Figure 31.4 K space lines and numbering.

As a result of spatial encoding, spins are phase shifted along one axis of the image (see Chapter 29) and frequency shifted along the other (see Chapter 30). The system can now tell the individual spins apart by the number of times they pass across the receiver coil (frequency) and their position in the cycle as they do so (phase). However, in order to translate the information obtained from the encoding process into an image, the frequencies within the signal must be digitized through a process called **analogue to digital conversion** or **ADC** and stored as data points in an area of the array processor known as **K space**.

The image consists of a **field of view (FOV)** that relates to the amount of anatomy covered. The FOV can be square or rectangular, and is divided up into **pixels** or picture elements. The pixels exist within a two-dimensional grid or **matrix** into which the system maps each individual signal. When the slice thickness is considered, a three-dimensional **voxel** is produced (Figure 31.1).

The number of pixels within the FOV depends on the number of frequency samples and phase encodings performed. Each pixel is allocated a signal intensity depending on the signal amplitude, with a distinct frequency and phase shift value. This is performed via by a mathematical process known as **fast Fourier transform** or **FFT**. In its raw data form, the frequency of each signal is plotted against time, i.e. the signal is measured in relation to its amplitude over a period of time. During FFT the system converts this raw data so that the signal amplitude is measured relative to its frequency. This enables the creation of an image, where each pixel is allocated a signal intensity corresponding to the amplitude of signal originating from anatomy at the position of each pixel in the matrix (Figure 31.2).

Before FFT can be performed, however, data points must be stored in K space. K space is a spatial frequency domain, i.e. where information about the frequency of a signal and where it comes from in the patient is collected and stored. As frequency is defined as phase change per unit time and is measured in radians, the unit of K space is **radians/cm**. K space does not correspond to the image, i.e. the top of K space does

not correspond with the top of the image. K space is merely an area where data is stored until the scan is over.

Each slice has its own area of K space, e.g. if 20 slices are selected there are 20 K-space areas in the array processor.

K space is rectangular and has two axes:
• The **frequency axis** of K space is horizontal, i.e. centred in the middle of the K space perpendicular to the phase axis.
• The **phase axis** of K space is vertical, perpendicular to the frequency axis (Figure 31.3).

K space consists of a series of horizontal **lines**, the number of which corresponds to the number of phase encodings performed (**phase matrix**). Each line is filled with a series of data points, the number of which corresponds to the number of frequency samples taken (**frequency matrix**). Every time the frequencies in an echo are sampled, the data collected is stored as data points in a line of K space.
• The lines **nearest** to the centre are called the **central** lines.
• The lines **farthest** from centre are called the **outer** lines.
• The **top half** of K space is termed **positive**.
• The **bottom half** of K space is termed **negative** (Figure 31.3).

The polarity of the phase gradient determines whether the positive or negative half of K space is filled. Positive gradient slopes fill lines in the positive half of K space, and negative gradients fill lines in the negative half (see Chapter 38).

Lines are numbered relative to the central horizontal axis, starting from the centre (low numbers) and moving out towards the outer areas of K space (high numbers). Lines in the top half are labelled positive, those in the bottom half, negative. The central lines of K space are always filled regardless of the phase matrix. For example, if 128-phase matrix is required, lines +64 to −64 are filled rather than lines +128 to 0. K-space lines are usually filled linearly, i.e. either from top to bottom, or from bottom to top (Figure 31.4).

K space is symmetrical about both axes, i.e. data in the right-hand side of K space is identical to that on the left, and data in the top half is identical to that in the bottom half. This is called **conjugate symmetry**.

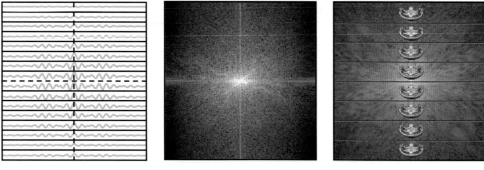

diagramatic   data   the chest of drawers

Figure 32.1 K space – the chest of drawers.

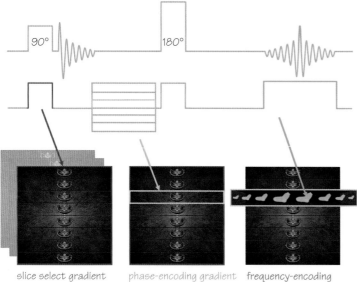

90°   180°

slice select gradient chooses which chest of drawers

phase-encoding gradient chooses which drawer to open

frequency-encoding gradient chooses where to put the socks

Figure 32.2 K space filling in spin echo.

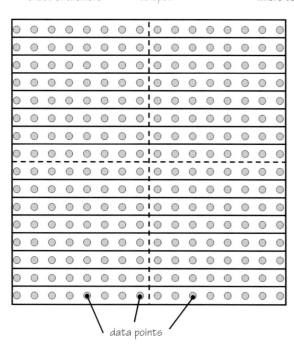

data points

Figure 32.3 Data points in K space.

The pulse sequence selected determines how K space is filled. Pulse sequences are defined as a series of RF pulses, gradient applications and intervening time periods. It is primarily the gradients that determine how K space is filled (see Chapter 38).

• The **slice select gradient** determines which slice is to be selected. As each slice as its own K-space area, the slice select gradient determines which K-space area is to be filled next.

• The **phase-encoding gradient** is the next gradient to be applied. The slope and polarity of this gradient determines which line of K space is to be filled. The polarity of this gradient determines whether a line in the top or bottom half of K space is filled (see Chapter 31). The slope of the phase gradient determines whether a central or outer line of K space is filled (see Chapter 33).

• The **frequency-encoding gradient** is switched on during the echo or signal. It is while this gradient is applied that frequencies from the echo are sampled, converted into data points and stored in each line of K space (see Chapter 35).

Learning point

K space is analogous to a chest of drawers as, just as a chest of drawers stores items such as socks in horizontal drawers, so does K space store data points in horizontal lines (Figure 32.1). Each K-space area, and therefore each slice selected, represents a different chest of drawers.

Imagine that there is a pile containing nearly 2 million socks in the middle of a room surrounded by 30 chest of drawers, each containing 256 drawers. Your task is to place 256 socks into each drawer in every drawer of every chest of drawers. That would be quite a task, and to perform it efficiently you would have to fill each drawer methodically in a particular order. How do you think you could do this?

This is like the system computer having nearly 2 million data points from 30 slices (each slice having a phase and frequency matrix of 256) that it must place into 30 different K-space areas. Pulse sequences enable the system to perform this task methodically and efficiently. The gradients applied in a sequence determine how this may be done thus (see Chapter 38):

• the slice select gradient chooses which chest of drawers to walk up to (1–30);
• the phase-encoding gradient selects which drawer to open (1–256);
• the frequency-encoding gradient is on when 256 socks are put into this drawer from one side to the other (Figure 32.2).

This is why each gradient is applied in this order in a sequence as it is obviously necessary to walk up to a chest of drawers first, then open a drawer and then place socks within the drawer. Remember in this analogy that socks are data points and each chest of drawers represents a slice.

Once a particular drawer is filled, the **same** drawer in another chest of drawers is filled with socks. This requires the slice select gradient to be switched on again to excite another slice and hence walk up to another chest of drawers. The phase-encoding gradient must then be switched on again to the **same** slope and polarity to fill the **same** drawer in this chest of drawers. The frequency-encoding gradient is then switched on again so that 256 data points (socks) can be placed in the drawer.

This sequence is continued until the **same** drawer is filled in every chest of drawers (e.g. the top drawer of chests 1 to 30). Once all the top drawers are filled in every chest of drawers, the TR period is repeated by applying another excitation pulse to the first slice. However, in this TR period a **different** drawer is filled to that in the first TR period. To do this the slope of the phase-encoding gradient is changed to open the next drawer down from the top. The sequence is continued, the same drawer being filled in each chest of drawers in a particular TR period. Every TR the slope of the phase gradient is changed to open the next drawer down, until all the drawers of all the chest of drawers are filled with socks (data points). The number of data points in each row or drawer corresponds to the frequency matrix selected. The number of data points in each column corresponds to the phase matrix and to the number of drawers in each chest of drawers (Figure 32.3). Using this example there would be a total of 1,966,080 socks or data points stored ($256 \times 256 \times 30$).

This is only one way in which the drawers may be filled; there are many other permutations (see Chapter 37).

33 K space filling and signal amplitude

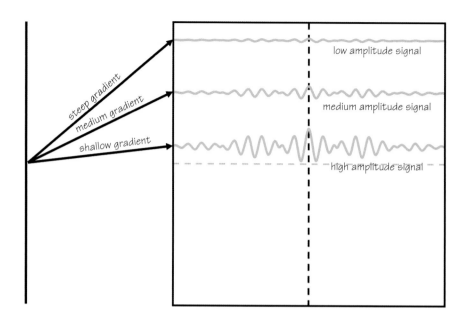

Figure 33.1 *Phase gradient amplitude vs signal amplitude.*

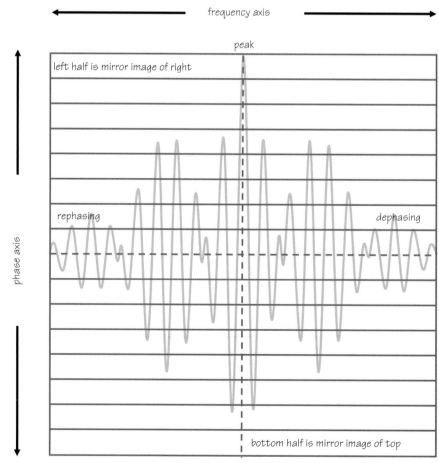

Figure 33.2 *Frequency encoding vs signal amplitude.*

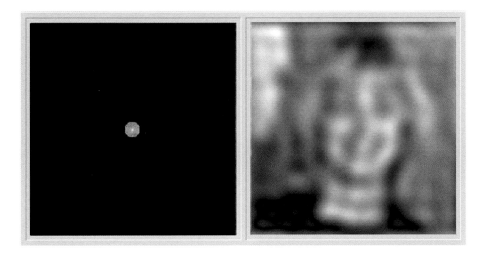

Figure 33.3 Image using central K space data points only.

Phase data

The **central** lines of K space are filled with data produced after the application of **shallow** phase-encoding gradient slopes. The **outer** lines of K space are filled with data produced after the application of the **steep** phase-encoding gradient slopes. The lines in between the central and outer portions are filled with the intermediate phase-encoding slopes.

Shallow phase-encoding slopes do not produce a large phase shift along their axis. Therefore rephasing of magnetic moments by an RF pulse or a gradient is more efficient, as the inherent phase shift after phase encoding is small. **The resultant signal therefore has a large amplitude** as a high proportion of the spins are rephased by an RF pulse or a gradient to produce an echo.

Steep phase-encoding slopes produce a large phase shift along their axis. Therefore rephasing of magnetic moments is less efficient because the inherent phase shift after phase encoding is great. **The resultant signal has a small amplitude** as a small proportion of the spins are rephased by an RF pulse or a gradient to produce an echo (Figure 33.1).

Therefore the central lines of K space which are filled when shallow phase gradients are applied, contain data points that represent high signal amplitude.

Frequency data

Frequencies sampled from the signal are mapped into K space relative to the frequency axis. The centre of the echo represents the maximum signal amplitude as all the magnetic moments are in phase at this point, whereas magnetic moments are either rephasing or dephasing on either side of the peak of the echo, and therefore the signal amplitude here is less. The amplitude of frequencies sampled is mapped relative to the central vertical axis, so that the centre of the echo is placed over this axis. The rephasing and dephasing portions of the echo are mapped to the left and the right and, as the echo is symmetrical about this axis, frequency profiles in the left half of K space are identical to those on the right (Figure 33.2).

Therefore the central points in K space contain data points that represent the highest signal amplitude both in terms of phase data and frequency data. Therefore if an image is produced solely from these data points it has a high signal to noise ratio (see Chapter 40) and contrast. However it also has poor resolution (see Chapter 34) (Figure 33.3).

K space filling and spatial resolution

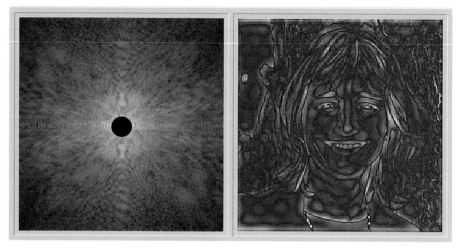

Figure 34.1 Image using the outer K-space data points only.

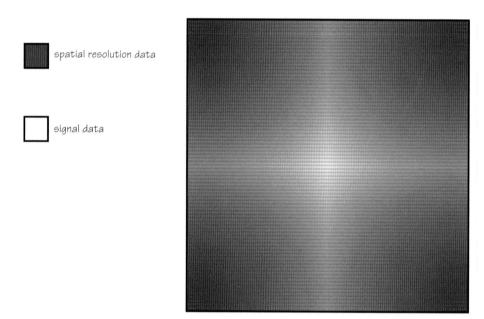

spatial resolution data

signal data

Figure 34.2 K space and signal and resolution data.

The outer lines of K space contain data produced after steep phase-encoding gradient slopes, and are only filled when many phase encodings have been performed. The number of phase encodings performed determines the number of pixels in the FOV along the phase-encoding axis. When a large number of phase encodings are performed, there are more pixels in the FOV along the phase axis and therefore each pixel is smaller. If the FOV is fixed, pixels of smaller dimensions result in an image with a high spatial resolution, i.e. two points within the image can be distinguished more easily when the pixels are small (see Chapter 42). In addition, as the amplitude of the phase-encoding gradient slope increases, the degree of phase shift along the gradient also increases. Two points adjacent to each other have a different phase value and can therefore be differentiated from each other. Therefore data collected after steep phase-encoding gradient slopes produces greater spatial resolution in the image than when using shallow phase-encoding slopes.

Therefore the outer points in K space, particularly in the vertical axis, contain data points that represent the best resolution. If an image is produced solely from these data points it has high spatial resolution (see Chapter 42). However, it also has poor signal and contrast (see Chapter 33) (Figure 34.1).

Summary
• The outer lines of K space contain data with high spatial resolution as they are filled by steep phase-encoding gradient slopes.
• The central lines of K space contain data with low spatial resolution as they are filled by shallow phase-encoding gradient slopes.
• The central portion of K space contains data that has high signal amplitude and low spatial resolution.
• The outer portion of K space contains data that has high spatial resolution and low signal amplitude (Figure 34.2).

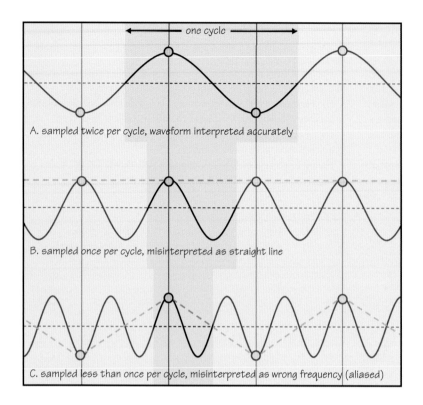

A. sampled twice per cycle, waveform interpreted accurately

B. sampled once per cycle, misinterpreted as straight line

C. sampled less than once per cycle, misinterpreted as wrong frequency (aliased)

Figure 35.1 The Nyquist theorem.

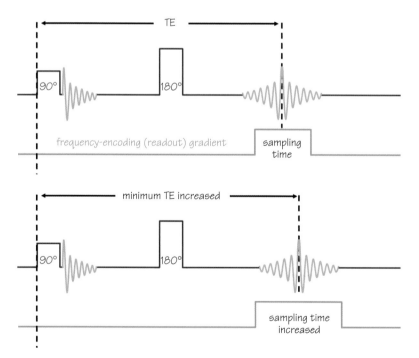

Figure 35.2 Sampling time and the TE.

The application of RF excitation pulses and gradients produces a range of different frequencies within the echo. This is called the **receive bandwidth** as a range of frequencies are being received. All of these frequencies must be sampled by the system in order to produce an accurate image from the data. The magnitude of the frequency encoding gradient, along with the receive bandwidth, determines the size of the FOV in the frequency encoding direction i.e. the distance across the patient into which the frequencies within the echo must fit.

Every time frequencies are sampled, data is stored in a line of K space. This is called a **data point**. The number of data points in each line of K space corresponds to the frequency matrix (e.g. 256, 512, 1024).

After the scan is over, the computer looks at the data points in K space and mathematically converts information in each data point into a frequency. From this the image is formed. As the frequency-encoding gradient is always applied during the sampling of data from the echo, it is often called the **readout gradient** (although the gradient is not collecting the data, the computer is doing this).

• The time available to the system to sample frequencies in the signal is called the **sampling time**.
• The rate at which frequencies are sampled is called the **sampling rate**.
• The sampling rate is determined by the receive bandwidth. If the receive bandwidth is 32 kHz this means that frequencies are sampled at a rate of 32,000 times per second.
• The **Nyquist theorem** that states that the sampling rate must be at least twice the frequency of the highest frequency in the echo. If this does not occur, data points collected in K space do not accurately reflect all frequencies present in the signal.

In order to produce an accurate image, the frequencies derived from the data points must look like the original frequencies in the signal. If the sampling rate frequency only matches the highest frequency present in the echo, only one data point is collected per cycle. This means that there is insufficient data to accurately reproduce all the original frequencies. If the sampling rate frequency obeys the Nyquist theorem and samples at twice the highest frequency in the echo, then there are sufficient data points to accurately reproduce the original frequencies (Figure 35.1).

There is a relationship between the receive bandwidth and the frequency matrix selected. Enough data points must be collected to achieve the required frequency matrix with a particular receive bandwidth.

Changing the receive bandwidth
Frequency matrix 256
If the frequency matrix is 256, then 256 data points must be collected and laid out in each line of K space. The receive bandwidth determines the number of times per second a data point is collected. The sampling time must be long enough therefore to collect the required number of data points with the receive bandwidth selected.

For example:
• **Receive bandwidth 32,000 Hz** (32,000 samples/sec)

sampling rate = one sample every 0.03125 ms

256 data points to be collected

$0.0325 \times 256 = 8$ ms

sampling time must therefore = 8 ms

• **Receive bandwidth 16,000 Hz** (16,000 samples/sec)

sampling rate = one sample every 0.0625 ms

only 128 data points can be collected at this rate in 8 ms

to acquire 256 data points sampling time must therefore = 16 ms

Therefore, if the receive bandwidth is reduced without altering any other parameter, there are insufficient data points to produce a 256-frequency matrix.

As the sampling rate is not changed, the sampling time must be increased to collect the necessary 256 points. As the echo is usually centred in the middle of the sampling window, the minimum TE increases as the sampling time increases (Figure 35.2).

Changing the frequency matrix
Frequency matrix 512
If the frequency matrix is 512, then 512 data points must be collected and laid out in each line of K space. The number of frequencies that occur during the sampling time is determined by the receive bandwidth and the sampling time.

For example:
• **Receive bandwidth 32,000 Hz** (32,000 samples/sec)

sampling rate = one sample every 0.03125 ms

sampling time = 8 ms

256 data points collected = frequency matrix 256

Therefore, if the frequency matrix is increased without altering any other parameter, there are insufficient data points to produce a 512-frequency matrix.

As the sampling rate is not changed, the sampling time must be increased to permit acquisition of 512 data points in each line of K space during the sampling window. As the echo is usually centred in the middle of the sampling window, the minimum TE increases as the sampling time increases.

• **Therefore either increasing the frequency matrix or reducing the receive bandwidth increases the minimum TE.**

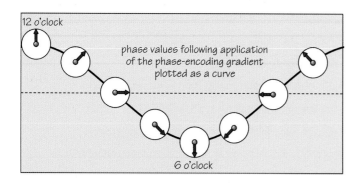

Figure 36.1 The phase curve.

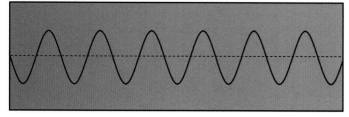

Figure 36.2 Different pseudofrequencies.

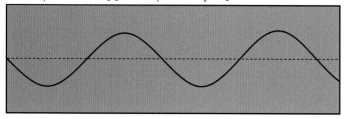

Figure 36.3 Columns and rows in K space.

A certain value of phase shift is obtained according to the slope of the phase-encoding gradient. The slope of the phase-encoding gradient determines which line of K space is filled with the data in each TR period. In order to fill out different lines of K space, the slope of the phase-encoding gradient is altered after each TR. If the slope of the phase-encoding gradient is not altered, the same line of K space is filled in all the time. In order to finish the scan or acquisition, all the selected lines of K space must be filled. The number of lines of K space that are filled is determined by the number of different phase-encoding slopes that are applied (see Chapter 32).

- Phase matrix = 128, 128 lines of K space are filled to complete the scan.
- Phase matrix = 256, 256 lines of K space are filled to complete the scan.

The slope of the phase-encoding gradient determines the magnitude of the phase shift between two points in the patient. **Steep** slopes produce a **large phase difference** between two points, whereas **shallow** slopes produce **small phase shifts** between the same two points. The system cannot measure phase directly; it can only measure frequency. The system therefore converts the phase shift into frequency by creating a waveform created by combining all the phase values associated with a certain phase shift. This waveform has a certain frequency or pseudofrequency (as it has been indirectly obtained) (Figure 36.1).

In order to fill a different line of K space, a different pseudofrequency must be obtained. If a different pseudofrequency is not obtained, the same line of K space is filled over and over again. To create a different pseudofrequency, a different phase shift must be produced by the phase-encoding gradient. The phase-encoding gradient is therefore switched on to a different amplitude or slope, to produce a different phase shift value. Therefore, the change in phase shift created by the altered phase-encoding gradient slope results in a waveform with a different pseudofrequency (Figure 36.2).

Every TR, each slice is frequency encoded (resulting in the same frequency shift), and phase encoded with a different slope of phase-encoding gradient to produce a different pseudofrequency. Once all the lines of selected K space have been filled with data points, acquisition of data is complete and the scan is over. The acquired data held in K space is now converted into an image via FFT (see Chapter 31) (Figure 36.3).

2D sequential
acquisition

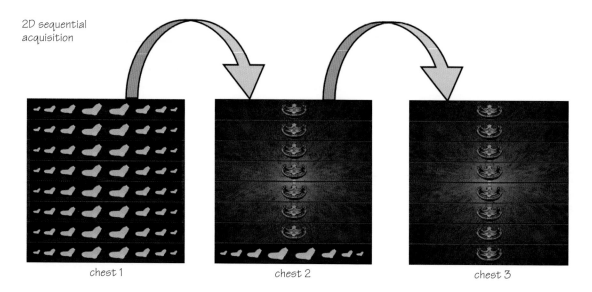

chest 1 chest 2 chest 3

2D volumetric
acquisition

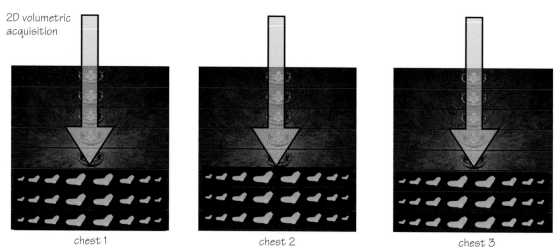

chest 1 chest 2 chest 3

Figure 37.1 Data acquisition methods.

In conventional data acquisition:

the scan time = TR × phase matrix × number of signal averages (NSA)

TR

In standard acquisition, every TR, each slice is frequency encoded (resulting in the same frequency shift), and phase encoded with a different slope of phase-encoding gradient to produce a different pseudo-frequency. Different lines in K space are therefore filled after every TR. Once all the lines of selected K space have been filled, acquisition of data is complete and the scan is over (see Chapter 32).

Phase matrix

The phase-encoding gradient slope is altered every TR and is applied to each selected slice in order to phase encode it. After each phase encode a different line of K space is filled. The number of phase-encoding steps therefore affects the length of the scan.

- **128** phase encodings selected (phase matrix = 128), **128 lines** are filled.
- **256** phase encodings selected (phase matrix = 256), **256 lines** are filled.
  As one phase encoding is performed each TR (to each slice):
- **128** phase encodings requires **128 × TR** to complete the scan.
- **256** phase encodings requires **256 × TR** to complete the scan.
- If the TR is 1 sec (1000 ms) the scan takes 128 s (if 128 phase encodings are performed) and 256 s (if 256 phase encodings are performed).

Number of signal averages (NSA)

The signal can be sampled more than once after the same slope of phase-encoding gradient. Doing so will fill each line of K space more than once. The number of times each signal is sampled after the same slope of phase-encoding gradient is usually called the **number of signal averages (NSA)** or **the number of excitations (NEX)**. The higher the NSA, the more data that is stored in each line of K space. As there is more data stored in each line of K space, the amplitude of signal at each frequency and phase shift is greater (see Chapter 40).

Types of acquisition

Three-dimensional volumetric sequential acquisitions acquire all the data from slice 1 and then go onto acquire all the data from slice 2, and so on (all the lines in K space are filled for slice 1 and then all the lines of K space are filled for slice 2, etc.). The slices are therefore displayed as they are acquired.

Two-dimensional volumetric acquisitions, fill one line of K space for slice 1, and then go onto to fill the **same** line of K space for slice 2, and so on. When this line has been filled for all the slices, the next line of K space is filled for slice 1, 2, 3, etc. (Figure 37.1). This is the type of acquisition discussed in Chapter 32.

Three-dimensional volumetric acquisition (volume imaging) acquires data from an entire volume of tissue, rather than in separate slices. The excitation pulse is not slice selective, and the whole prescribed imaging volume is excited. At the end of the acquisition the volume or slab is divided into discrete locations or partitions by the slice select gradient that, when switched on, separates the slices according to their phase value along the gradient. This process is called **slice encoding**. As slice encoding is similar to phase encoding, the number of slice locations increase the scan time proportionally, e.g. for 72 slice locations the scan time = TR × phase matrix × NSA × 72. This increases the scan time significantly compared to other types of acquisitions and therefore volume imaging should only be performed with fast sequences. However, many thin slices can be obtained without a slice gap, thereby increasing resolution.

38 K space traversal and pulse sequences

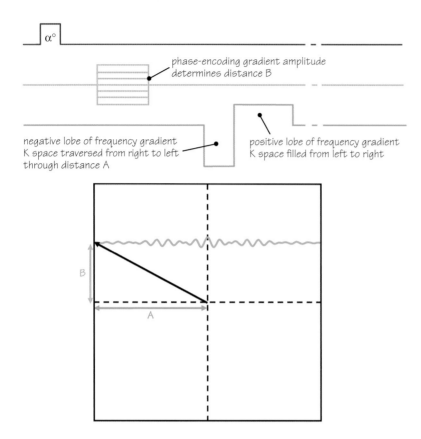

phase-encoding gradient amplitude determines distance B

negative lobe of frequency gradient
K space traversed from right to left
through distance A

positive lobe of frequency gradient
K space filled from left to right

Figure 38.1 K space traversal in gradient echo.

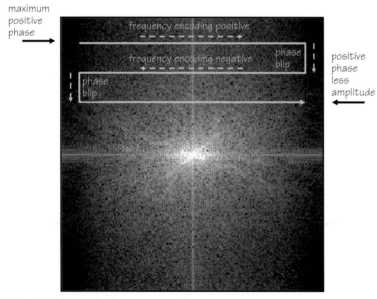

Figure 38.2 Single-shot K space traversal.

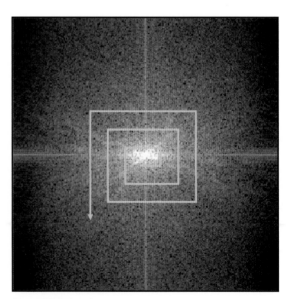

Figure 38.3 Spiral K space traversal.

The way in which K space is traversed and filled depends on a combination of the polarity and amplitude of both the frequency-encoding and phase-encoding gradients.

- The amplitude of the **frequency**-encoding gradient determines how far to **the left and right** K space is traversed and this in turn determines the size of the FOV in the frequency direction of the image.
- The amplitude of the **phase**-encoding gradient determines how far **up and down** a line of K space is filled and in turn determines the phase matrix.

The polarity of each gradient defines the direction travelled through K space as follows:

- **frequency**-encoding gradient **positive**, K space traversed **from left to right**;
- **frequency**-encoding gradient **negative**, K space traversed **from right to left**;
- **phase**-encoding gradient **positive**, fills **top** half of K space;
- **phase**-encoding gradient **negative**, fills **bottom** half of K space.

K space traversal in gradient echo

In a gradient echo sequence the frequency-encoding gradient switches negatively to forcibly dephase the FID and then positively to rephase and produce a gradient echo (see Chapter 17).

- When the frequency-encoding gradient is negative, K space is traversed from right to left. The starting point of K-space filling is usually at the centre as this is the effect RF excitation pulse has on K-space traversal. Therefore K space is initially traversed from the centre to the left, to a distance (A) that depends on the amplitude of the negative lobe of the frequency-encoding gradient (Figure 38.1).
- The phase encode in this example is positive and therefore a line in the top half of K space is filled. The amplitude of this gradient determines the distance travelled (B). The larger the amplitude of the phase gradient, the higher up in K space the line that is filled with data from the echo. Therefore the combination of the phase gradient and the negative lobe of the frequency gradient determines at what point in K space data storage begins.
- The frequency-encoding gradient is then switched positively and, during its application, data points are laid out in a line of K space. As the frequency-encoding gradient is positive, data points are placed in a line

of K space from left to right. The distance travelled depends on the amplitude of the positive lobe of the gradient, which in turn determines the size of the FOV in the frequency direction of the image.

- If the phase gradient is negative then a line in the bottom half of K space is filled in exactly the same manner.

K space traversal in spin echo

K space traversal in spin echo sequences is more complex as the 180° RF pulse causes the point to which K space has been traversed to be flipped to the mirror point on the opposite side of K space both left to right and top to bottom. Therefore, in spin echo, the frequency gradient configurations necessary to reach the left side of K space and begin data collection are two identical lobes on either side of the 180° RF pulse.

K space traversal in single shot

Filling K space in single shot imaging involves rapidly switching the frequency-encoding gradient from positive to negative; positively to fill a line of K space from left to right and negatively to fill a line from right to left. As the frequency-encoding gradient switches its polarity so rapidly it is said to oscillate.

The phase gradient also has to switch on and off rapidly. The first application of the phase gradient is maximum positive to fill the top line. The next application (to encode the next echo) is still positive but its amplitude is slightly less, so that the next line down is filled. This process is repeated until the centre of K space is reached when the phase gradient switches negatively to fill the bottom lines. The amplitude is gradually increased until maximum negative polarity is achieved filling the bottom line of K space. This type of gradient switching is called **blipping** (Figure 38.2).

K space traversal in spiral imaging

A more complex type of K space traversal is spiral. In this example both the readout and the phase gradient switch their polarity rapidly and oscillate. In this spiral form of K space traversal, not only does the frequency-encoding gradient oscillate to fill lines from left to right and then right to left, but as K space filling begins at the centre, the phase gradient must also oscillate to fill a line in the top half followed by a line in the bottom half (Figure 38.3).

39 Alternative K-space filling techniques

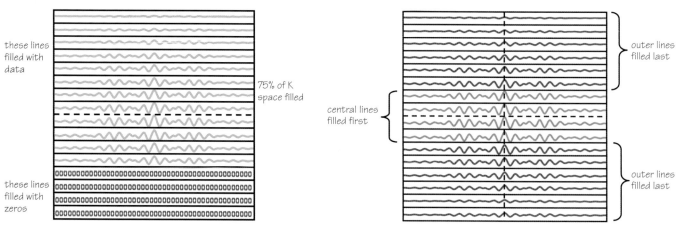

these lines filled with data

75% of K space filled

these lines filled with zeros

Figure 39.1 Partial Fourier.

outer lines filled last

central lines filled first

outer lines filled last

Figure 39.2 Centric K space filling.

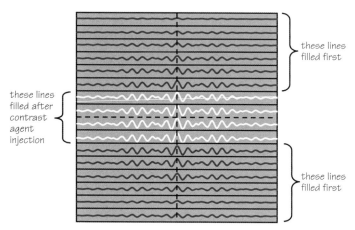

these lines filled first

these lines filled after contrast agent injection

these lines filled first

Figure 39.3 Keyhole imaging.

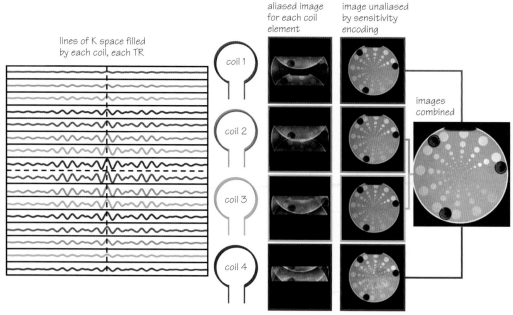

lines of K space filled by each coil, each TR

aliased image for each coil element

image unaliased by sensitivity encoding

coil 1

coil 2

coil 3

coil 4

images combined

Figure 39.4 Parallel imaging.

Partial or fractional averaging

• Partial averaging exploits the symmetry of K space. As long as at least 60% of the lines of K space are filled during the acquisition, the system has enough data to produce an image.

• The scan produced is reduced proportionally.

• For example, if only 75% of K space is filled, only 75% of the phase encodings selected need to be performed to complete the scan, and the remaining lines are filled with zeros. The scan time is therefore reduced by 25% but less data is acquired so the image has lower SNR (see Chapter 40) (Figure 39.1).

Rectangular FOV (see Chapter 42)

• The incremental step between each line of K space is inversely proportional to the FOV in the phase direction as a percentage of the FOV in the frequency direction. In rectangular FOV the size of the incremental step between each line is increased.

• The outermost lines of K space are filled to maintain resolution (e.g. 256 × 256, ± 128 lines filled).

• If the incremental step between each line is increased then fewer lines are filled.

• The scan time is reduced as fewer lines are filled.

• The size of the FOV in the phase direction decreases relative to frequency and a rectangular FOV results.

Anti-aliasing/Oversampling (see Chapter 48)

• The incremental step between each line of K space is inversely proportional to the FOV in the phase direction as a percentage of the FOV in the frequency direction. In anti-aliasing, the incremental step between each line is decreased.

• The outermost lines of K space are filled to maintain resolution (e.g. 256 × 256, ± 128 lines filled).

• As more lines are filled, oversampling of data occurs so there is less likelihood of phase duplication between anatomy outside the FOV and that inside the FOV in the phase direction.

• The scan time increases as more lines are filled. The NSA is either automatically reduced to maintain the original scan time, or some systems maintain the original NSA and the scan time increases proportionally.

• The size of the FOV in the phase direction is increased, making it less likely that anatomy will exist outside a larger FOV thereby reducing aliasing. On some systems the extended FOV is discarded. On others it is maintained, thereby reducing resolution.

Centric imaging

In this technique the central lines of K space are filled before the outer lines to maximize signal and contrast. This is important in sequences such as fast gradient echo where signal amplitude is compromised (see Chapter 24) (Figure 39.2).

Keyhole imaging

Keyhole techniques are often used in dynamic imaging after administration of gadolinium. The outer lines are filled before gadolinium arrives in the imaging volume. When it is in the area of interest, only the central lines are filled. Then data from both the outer lines and central lines are used to construct the image. In this way resolution is maintained but, as only the central lines are filled when gadolinium is in the imaging volume, temporal resolution is increased during this period. In addition, as the central lines are filled during this time, signal and contrast data are acquired thereby enhancing the visualization of gadolinium (see Chapter 53) (Figure 39.3).

Parallel imaging

In this technique multiple receiver coils or channels are used during the sequence. Each coil or channel delivers data to their own unique lines of K space and hence K space may be filled faster than if these coils are not used. For example, if two coils or channels are used, one coil supplies data to all the odd lines of K space and the other to all the even lines (see Chapter 57). During each TR period two lines are acquired together, one from coil 1 and the other from coil 2. Therefore the scan time is halved. The number of coils or channels is usually called the reduction factor and, unlike TSE (which also fills multiple lines of K space per TR), can be used with any type of sequence.

An image is produced for each coil. As each coil does not supply data to every line of K space, the incremental step between each line for each coil is increased. As a result, the FOV in the phase direction of each image is smaller than in the frequency direction and aliasing occurs. To remove the artefact, the system performs a calibration before each scan where it measures the signal intensity returned at certain distances away from each coil. This calibration or sensitivity profile is used to 'unwrap' each image. After this the data from each image from each coil are combined to produce a single image. This technique allows considerably shorter scan times and/or improved resolution, e.g. phase resolution of 512 in a scan time associated with a 256-phase matrix (Figure 39.4).

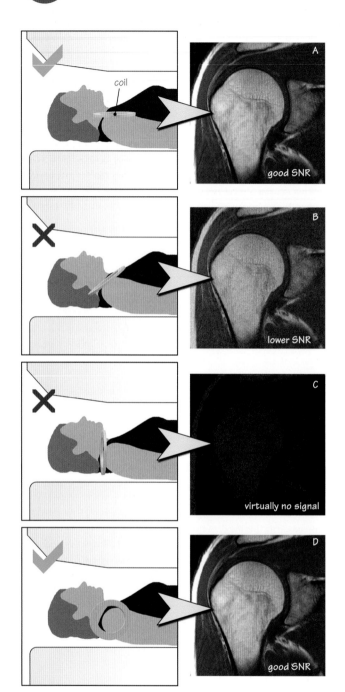

Figure 40.1 Coil placement versus SNR.

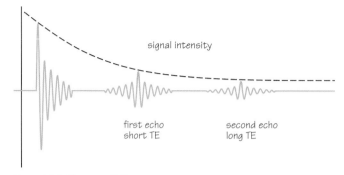

Figure 40.2 TE versus SNR.

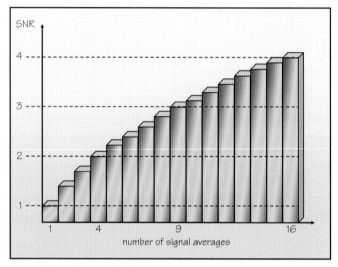

Figure 40.3 NSA versus SNR.

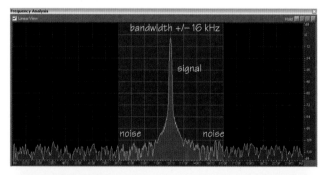

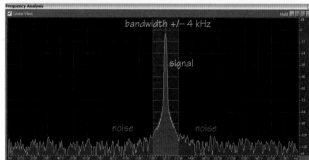

Figure 40.4 Receive bandwidth versus SNR.

Signal to noise ratio (SNR) is defined as the ratio of the amplitude of the MR signal to the average amplitude of the background noise. The **MR signal** is the voltage induced in the receiver coil by the precession of the NMV in the transverse plane. It occurs at specific frequencies and time intervals (TE). **Noise** is the undesired signal resulting from the MR system, the environment and the patient. It occurs at all frequencies and randomly in time and space. To increase the SNR usually requires increasing the signal relative to the noise. Some of the parameters that affect SNR are as follows.

Proton density

Some structures contain tissues such as fat, muscle and bone that have a high proton density. On the other hand, the chest contains mainly air-filled lung spaces, vessels and very little dense tissue. When scanning areas with a low proton density it is likely that measures to boost the SNR will be required.

Coil type and position

Small coils provide good local SNR but have a small coverage. Large coils provide much larger coverage but result in lower SNR. A good compromise is to use a phased array coil that uses multiple small coils which provide good SNR, and the data from these are combined to produce an image with good coverage (see Chapter 57).

The positioning of the receiver coil is also important. In order to receive maximum signal, receiver coils must be placed in the transverse plane perpendicular to the main field. In a superconducting system this means placing the coil over, under or to the side of the area being examined. Orientation of the coil perpendicular to the table results in zero signal generation (Figure 40.1).

TR

The TR determines how much the longitudinal magnetization recovers between excitation pulses and how much is available to be flipped into the transverse plane in the next TR period (see Chapter 7). Using short TRs, very little longitudinal magnetization recovers, so only a small amount of transverse magnetization is created and therefore results in an image with poor SNR. Increasing the TR until all tissues have recovered their longitudinal magnetization improves the SNR as more longitudinal magnetization (and therefore more transverse magnetization) is created. Although short TRs are required for T1 weighting, reducing this parameter too much may severely compromise SNR.

TE

The TE determines how much dephasing of transverse magnetization occurs between the excitation pulse and the echo. At short TEs, as very little transverse magnetization has dephased, the signal amplitude and therefore the SNR of the image is high. Increasing the TE reduces the SNR as more transverse magnetization dephases (Figure 40.2). Although long TEs are required for T2 weighting, increasing this parameter too much compromises the SNR (see Chapter 8).

Flip angle

The size of the flip angle determines how much of the longitudinal magnetization is converted into transverse magnetization by the excitation pulse. With a large flip angle, all available longitudinal magnetization is converted into transverse magnetization, whereas with small flip angles only a proportion of the longitudinal magnetization is converted to transverse magnetization. The flip angle is commonly varied in gradient echo sequences where a low flip angle is required for T2* and proton density weighted imaging (see Chapter 17). However they also result in images with low SNR and hence measures may have to be taken to improve it.

Number of signal averages (NSA)

This parameter determines the number of times frequencies in the signal are sampled after the same slope of phase encoding gradient (see Chapter 37). Increasing the NSA increases the signal collected. However noise is also sampled. As noise occurs at all frequencies and randomly, doubling the NSA only increases the SNR by the square of root of 2. Because of this relationship, the benefits of increasing the SNR as the NSA increases are reduced but the scan times increases proportionally (Figure 40.3).

Receive bandwidth

This is the range of frequencies sampled during readout (see Chapter 35). Reducing the receive bandwidth reduces the proportion of noise sampled relative to signal (Figure 40.4). Reducing the receive bandwidth is a very effective way of boosting the SNR. However reducing the bandwidth:
• increases the minimum TE so this technique is not suitable for T1 or PD imaging (see Chapter 35);
• increases an artefact known as chemical shift (see Chapter 45).

Despite these tradeoffs, reduced receive bandwidths should be used when a short TE is not required (T2 weighting) and when fat is not present. An example is an examination when fat is suppressed in conjunction with T2 weighting, e.g. T2 TSE and STIR (Figure 16.4).

The FOV, matrix and slice thickness also affect the SNR (see Chapter 42), as does the field strength.

41 Contrast to noise ratio

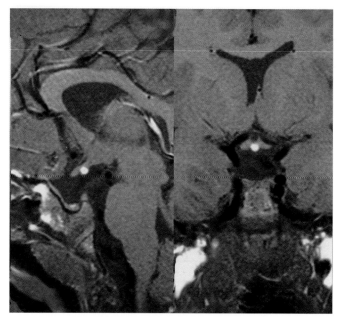

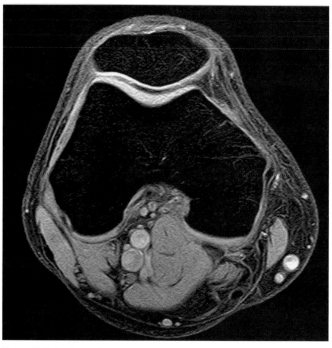

Figure 41.1 Sagittal (left) and coronal (right) T1 weighted image after contrast showing an ectopic posterior pituitary.

Figure 41.2 Axial slice from a 3D acquisition using chemical suppression.

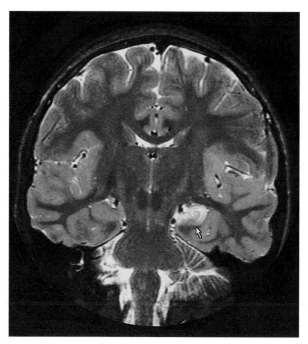

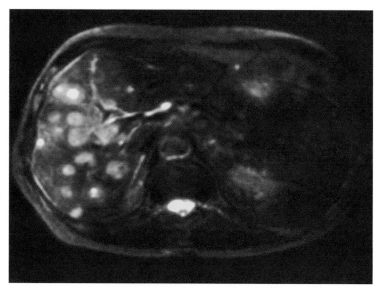

Figure 41.4 Axial T2 weighted image of the liver with chemical suppression. There is a good CNR between the liver lesions and normal liver using this technique although the overall image quality is poor.

Figure 41.3 Coronal T2 weighted image of the temporal lobes. The lesion (arrow) is clearly seen as a high signal with this weighting.

The **contrast to noise ratio** or **CNR** is defined as the difference in SNR between two adjacent areas. It is controlled by the same factors that affect SNR. The CNR is probably the most important image quality factor as the objective of any examination is to produce an image where pathology is clearly seen relative to normal anatomy. Visualization of a lesion increases if the CNR between it and surrounding anatomy is high. The CNR is increased by the following.

The administration of a contrast agent
Contrast agents such as gadolinium produce T1 shortening of lesions, especially those that cause a breakdown in the blood–brain barrier. As a result, enhancing tissue appears bright on T1 weighted images and therefore there is a good CNR between it and surrounding non-enhancing tissue (see Chapter 54) (Figure 41.1).

Magnetization transfer contrast
Magnetization transfer contrast (**MTC**) uses additional RF pulses to suppress hydrogen protons that are not free but bound to macro-molecules and cell membranes. These pulses are either applied at a frequency away from the Larmor frequency, where they are known as **off resonant**, or nearer to the centre frequency where they are known as **on resonant**. As a result of the application of these pulses, magnetization is transferred to the free protons suppressing the signal in certain types of tissue.

Chemical suppression techniques
These can be used to suppress signal from either fat or water. Fat suppression pulses are applied to the FOV prior to the excitation pulse, resulting in nulling of fat signal. As a consequence the CNR between lesions and surrounding normal tissue that contain fat is enhanced (Figure 41.2).

T2 weighting
T2 weighting is specifically used to increase the CNR between normal and abnormal tissue. Pathology is often bright on a T2 weighted image as it contains water. As a result pathology is more conspicuous than on T1 or PD weighted images (Figure 41.3).

Sometimes acquiring an image with good CNR means compromising other image quality factors. An example is in the liver when, in T1 weighted images, lesions and normal liver may be **isointense** (the same signal intensity). By acquiring fat-suppressed T2 weighted imaging, although SNR, spatial resolution and scan time are usually compromised because of the parameters selected, the CNR between lesions (bright) and normal liver (dark) is increased (Figure 41.4).

even matrix square field of view

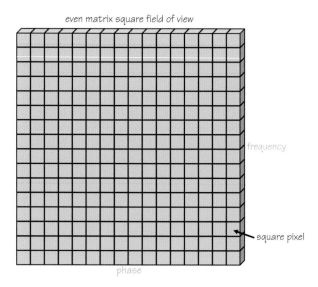

frequency

square pixel

phase

uneven matrix square field of view

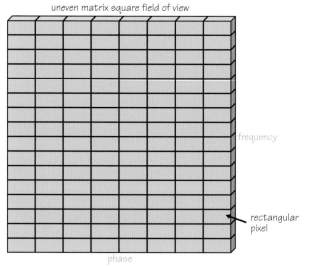

frequency

rectangular pixel

phase

Figure 42.1 Pixel size versus matrix size. Voxels are larger on the lower diagram, which results in a better SNR but poorer resolution than the upper diagram.

FOV 40 mm

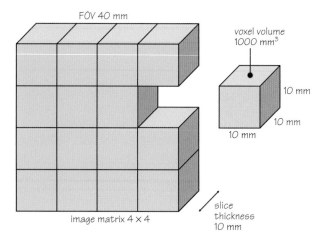

voxel volume 1000 mm³

10 mm
10 mm
10 mm

image matrix 4 × 4

slice thickness 10 mm

FOV 20 mm

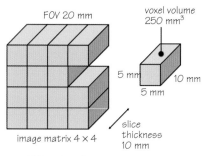

voxel volume 250 mm³

5 mm
10 mm
5 mm

image matrix 4 × 4

slice thickness 10 mm

Figure 42.2 FOV versus SNR and resolution.

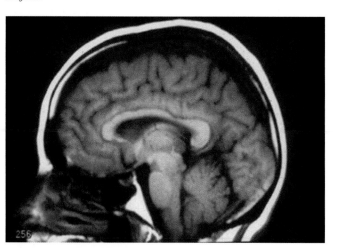

Figure 42.3 Sagittal image using a 10 mm slice thickness.

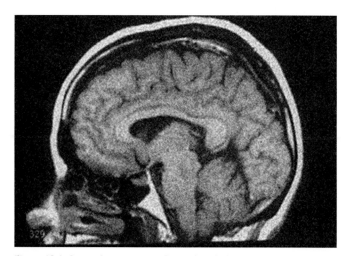

Figure 42.4 Sagittal image using a 3 mm slice thickness.

Spatial resolution is defined as the ability to distinguish between two points that are close together in the patient. It is entirely controlled by the size of the **voxel**.

- The imaging volume is divided into **slices**.
- Each slice displays an area of anatomy defined as the **field of view** or **FOV**.
- The FOV is divided into **pixels**, the size of which is controlled by the **matrix**.

The voxel is defined as the pixel area multiplied by the slice thickness (see Figure 31.1). Therefore the factors that affect the **voxel volume** are:

- slice thickness;
- FOV;
- matrix.

Voxel volume and SNR

The size of the voxel determines how much signal each voxel contains. Large voxels have higher signal than small ones because there are more spins in a large voxel to contribute to the signal. Therefore any setting of FOV, matrix size or slice thickness that results in large voxels leads to a higher SNR per voxel. However, as the voxels increase is size, resolution decreases. There is therefore a direct conflict between SNR and resolution in the geometry of the voxel.

Voxel volume and spatial resolution

Small voxels improve resolution as they increase the likelihood of two points, close together in the patient, being in separate voxels and therefore distinguishable from each other. Changing any dimension of the voxel changes the resolution but there is a direct trade-off with SNR.

Changing the matrix and SNR

This changes the dimension of each pixel along the frequency-encoding and phase-encoding axes depending on whether just one or both matrices are altered. If there are fewer pixels to map over the FOV, each pixel is larger. The SNR of each voxel therefore increases. Changing the phase matrix also changes scan time.

Changing the matrix and resolution

Changing the matrix alters the number of pixels that fit into the FOV. Therefore, as the matrix increases, pixel and therefore voxel size decrease. This increases resolution but reduces SNR. Changing the phase matrix also changes scan time (Figure 42.1).

Changing the FOV and SNR

The pixel (and therefore voxel) dimensions along each axis of the FOV change as the FOV changes. The SNR of each voxel increases by a factor of 4 because the dimensions of each pixel doubles along each axis of the FOV.

Changing the FOV and resolution

In Figure 42.2 an FOV of 40 mm, a non-representative matrix of 4×4 and a slice thickness of 10 mm are illustrated. This produces a voxel volume of 1000 mm^3. Halving the FOV to 20 mm reduces the voxel volume and therefore the SNR to a quarter of its original size, although spatial resolution is doubled along both the frequency and phase axes.

As reducing the FOV affects the size of the pixel along the both axes, the voxel volume is significantly reduced. Decreasing the FOV therefore has a drastic effect on SNR. Using a small FOV is appropriate when using small coils that boost local SNR, but should be employed with caution when using a large coil as SNR is severely compromised unless measures such as increasing the NSA are utilized.

Changing slice thickness and SNR

Changing the slice thickness changes the voxel volume along the dimension of the slice. Thick slices cover more of the patient's body tissue and therefore have more spinning protons within them. SNR therefore increases in proportion to increase in slice thickness.

Changing slice thickness and resolution

Changing the slice thickness changes the voxel volume proportionally and results in a change in both SNR and resolution. In Figure 42.3 a thick slice of 10 mm has been used. This image has good SNR but there is partial voluming leading to poor inslice resolution. In Figure 42.4 the slice thickness has been reduced to 3 mm. This image has poorer SNR due to a smaller voxel volume, and the inslice resolution has improved. However, as the pixel area has not changed, the image resolution is also unchanged.

Usually improving resolution requires a change in the phase matrix which leads to an increase in scan time. Sometimes, however, resolution can be increased without a corresponding increase in scan time. This can be done by:

- **Changing the frequency matrix only:** The frequency matrix does not affect scan time, but if increased, increases resolution.
- **Using asymmetric FOV:** This maintains the size of the FOV along the frequency axis but reduces the FOV in the phase direction (see Chapter 39). Therefore the resolution of a square FOV is maintained but the scan time is reduced in proportion to the reduction in the size of the FOV in the phase direction. This option is useful when anatomy fits into a rectangle, as in sagittal imaging of the pelvis.

43 Scan time

The scan time is determined by a combination of the TR, phase matrix and NSA.

scan time = TR × number of phase matrix × NSA

The longer a patient has to lie on the table the more likely it is that he/she will move and ruin the image (Figure 43.1). Therefore it is important to reduce scan times and make the patient as comfortable as possible. Good immobilization is also essential as a couple of minutes spent doing this may save you many more minutes in wasted sequences. To reduce scan times, the TR and/or the phase matrix and/or the NSA must be decreased (see Chapter 37). However there are trade-offs associated with this.

Reducing the TR
• Reduces the SNR because less longitudinal magnetization recovers during each TR period so that there is less to convert to transverse magnetization and therefore signal in the next TR period.
• Reduces the number of slices available in a single acquisition as there is less time to excite and rephase slices.
• Increases T1 weighting because the tissues are more likely to be saturated.

Reducing the phase matrix
• Reduces resolution because there are fewer pixels in the phase axis of the image and therefore two areas close together in the patient are less likely to be spatially separated. However, SNR is increased.

Reducing the NSA
• Reduces SNR because data from the signal is sampled and stored in K space less often.
• Increases some motion artefact because averaging of noise is less.
In two-dimensional sequences:

scan time = TR × number of phase matrix × NSA

In three-dimensional fast scan sequences:

scan time = TR × number of phase matrix × NSA × slice encodings

Three-dimensional scans apply a second phase-encoding gradient to select and excite each slice location so that scan time is also affected by the number of slice locations required in the volume (see Chapter 37).

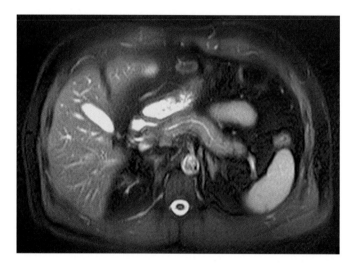

Figure 43.1 Axial T2 weighted image of the abdomen. The patient was unable to hold their breath for the duration of the selected scan time, and motion artefact has occurred.

44 Trade-offs

Table 44.1 The results of optimizing image quality

To optimize image	Adjusted parameter	consequence
Maximize SNR	↑ NEX	↑ scan time
	↓ matrix	↓ scan time
		↓ spatial resolution
	↑ slice thickness	↓ spatial resolution
	↓ receive bandwidth	↑ minimum TE
		↑ chemical shift
	↑ FOV	↓ spatial resolution
	↑ TR	↓ T1 weighting
		↑ number of slices
	↓ TE	↓ T2 weighting
Maximize spatial resolution (assuming a square FOV)	↓ slice thickness	↓ SNR
	↑ matrix	↓ SNR
		↑ scan time
	↓ FOV	↓ SNR
Minimize scan time		↑ T1 weighting
	↓ TR	↓ SNR
		↓ number of slices
	↓ phase encodings	↓ spatial resolution
		↑ SNR
	↓ NEX	↑ SNR
		↑ movement artefact
	↓ slice number in volume imaging	↓ SNR

Table 44.2 Parameters and their associated trade-offs

Parameter	Benefit	Limitation
TR increased	increased SNR increased number of slices	increased scan time decreased T1 weighting
TR decreased	decreased scan time increased T1 weighting	decreased SNR decreased number of slices
TE increased	increased T2 weighting	decreased SNR
TE decreased	increased SNR	decreased T2 weighting
NEX increased	increased SNR more signal averaging	direct proportional increase in scan time
NEX decreased	direct proportional decrease in scan time	decreased SNR less signal averaging
Slice thickness increased	increased SNR increased coverage of anatomy	decreased spatial resolution more partial voluming
Slice thickness decreased	increased spatial resolution reduced partial voluming	decreased SNR decreased coverage of anatomy
FOV increased	increased SNR increased coverage of anatomy	decreased spatial resolution decreased likelihood of aliasing
FOV decreased	increased spatial resolution increased likelihood of aliasing	decreased SNR decreased coverage of anatomy
Matrix increased	increased spatial resolution	increased scan time decreased SNR if pixel is small
Matrix decreased	decreased scan time increased SNR if pixel is large	decreased spatial resolution
Receive bandwidth increased	decrease in chemical shift decrease in minimum TE	decreased SNR
Receive bandwidth decreased	increased SNR	increase in chemical shift increase in minimum TE
Large coil	increased area of received signal	lower SNR sensitive to artefacts aliasing with small FOV
Small coil	increased SNR less sensitive to artefacts less prone to aliasing with a small FOV	decreased area of received signal

45 Chemical shift

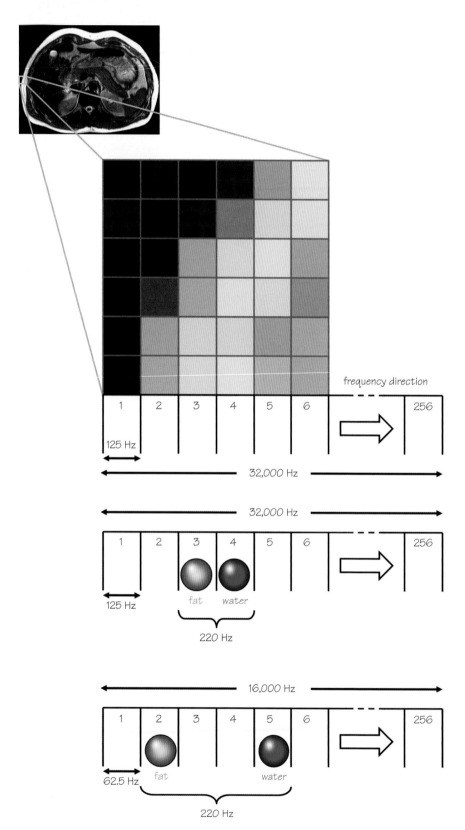

Figure 45.1 Chemical shift and the receive bandwidth.

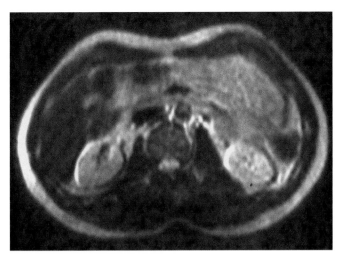

Figure 45.2 *Chemical shift artefact seen as a black band to the right of each kidney.*

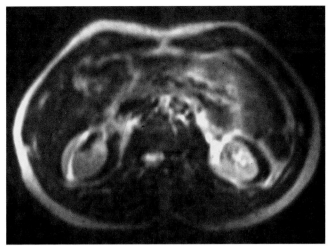

Figure 45.3 *Same patient as in Figure 45.2 but using a narrower receive bandwidth. The size of the chemical shift is reduced.*

Mechanism

Chemical shift artefact is a displacement of signal between fat and water along the frequency axis of the image. It is caused by the dissimilar chemical environments of fat and water that produces a precessional frequency difference between the magnetic moments of fat and water. In water, hydrogen is linked to oxygen; in fat it is linked to carbon. Due to the two different chemical environments, hydrogen in fat resonates at a lower frequency than in water. There is therefore a **frequency shift** inherently present between fat and water. Its magnitude depends on the magnetic field strength of the system and significantly increases at higher field strengths.

The **receive bandwidth** is one of the factors that controls chemical shift. It also controls SNR (see Chapter 40). The receive bandwidth determines the range of frequencies that must be mapped across pixels in the frequency direction of the FOV. It is selected to receive signal with frequencies slightly higher and lower than the centre frequency. It is usually measured in kHz (kilohertz). At 1.5 T with a receive bandwidth of ±16 kHz on either side of centre frequency, each pixel contains a range of frequencies, e.g. 125 Hz per pixel if the frequency matrix is 256, or 62.5 Hz per pixel if the frequency matrix is 512. If fat and water coexist in the same place in the patient, the frequency-encoding process maps fat hydrogen several Hz lower than water hydrogen into the image. They therefore appear in different pixels in the image despite coexisting in the patient. As the receive bandwidth is reduced, fewer frequencies are mapped across the same number of pixels. As a result, chemical shift artefact increases (Figure 45.1).

Appearance

Chemical shift artefact causes a signal void between areas of fat and water. An example is around the kidneys where the water-filled kidneys are surrounded by perirenal fat (Figure 45.3).

Remedy

- Scan with a low field-strength magnet.
- Remove either the fat or water signal by the use of STIR/chemical pre-saturation (see Chapters 16 and 49).
- Broaden the receive bandwidth (what is the trade-off?) (Figure 45.3).

46 Out-of-phase artefact

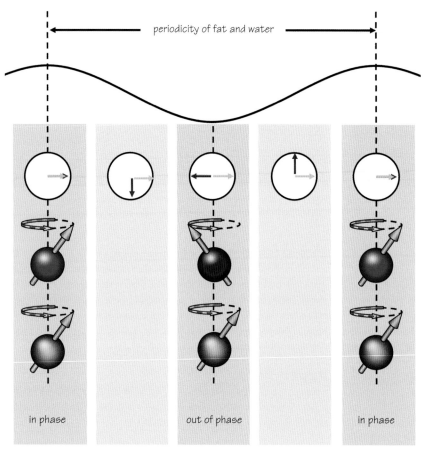

Figure 46.1 *The periodicity of fat and water.*

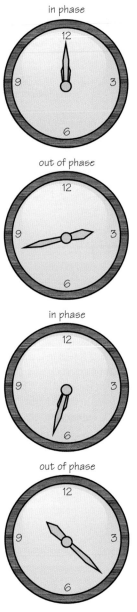

Figure 46.2 *The clock analogy.*

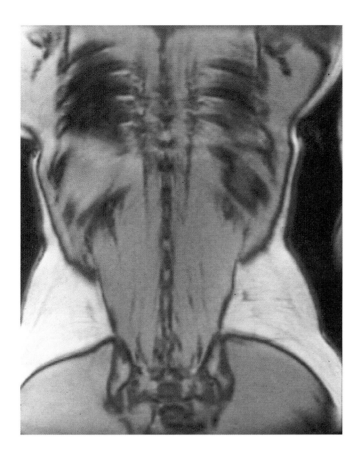

Figure 46.3 Out-of-phase artefact seen as a black line around the abdominal organs.

Mechanism

Out-of-phase artefact or **chemical misregistration** is caused by the difference in precessional frequency between fat and water that results in their magnetic moments being in phase with each other at certain times and out of phase at others (Figure 46.1). This is analogous to the hands on a clock which have different frequencies as they travel around the clock face. There are certain points when both hands are at the same phase and other times when they are not (Figure 46.2).

When the signals from both fat and water are out of phase, they cancel each other out so that signal loss results. If an image is produced when fat and water are out of phase, an artefact called **chemical misregistration** or **out-of-phase artefact** results. The time interval between fat and water being in phase is called the **periodicity**. This time depends on the frequency shift and therefore the field strength. At 1.5 T the periodicity is 4.2 ms. At lower field strengths the periodicity of fat and water is shorter and at higher field strengths it is longer.

Appearance

An out-of-phase image produces an asymmetrical edging effect (Figure 46.3). This artefact mainly occurs along the phase axis and causes a dark ring around structures that contain both fat and water. It is most prevalent in gradient echo sequences because gradient rephasing cannot compensate for the phase difference.

Remedy

• Use SE or FSE/TSE pulse sequences (which use RF rephasing pulses).
• Use a TE that matches the periodicity of fat and water so that the echo is generated when fat and water are in phase.
• The **Dixon technique** involves selecting a TE at half the periodicity so that fat and water are out of phase. In this way the signal from fat is reduced. This technique is mainly effective in areas where water and fat coexist in a voxel.

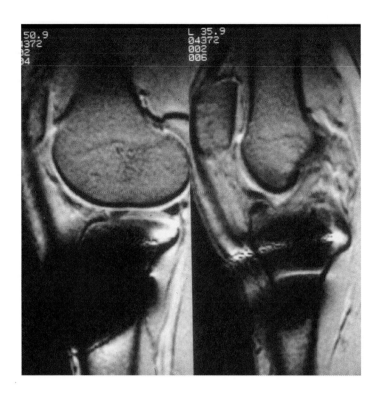

Figure 47.1 Sagittal GE imaging of the knee with metal screws in place. Magnetic susceptibility artefact is clearly seen.

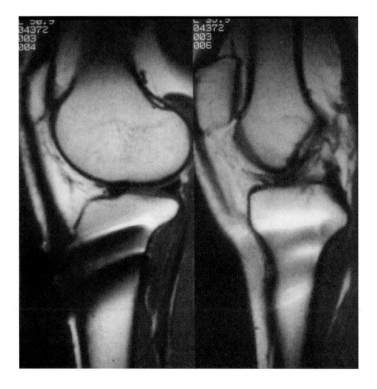

Figure 47.3 Same patient as in Figure 47.1 using a spin echo sequence. The artefact is reduced because RF rephasing corrects for differences in susceptibility between structures.

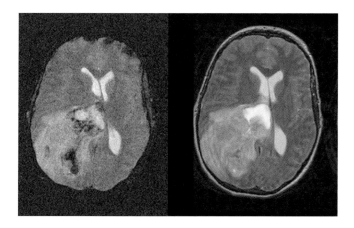

Figure 47.2 Axial GE T2* (left) and SE T2 (right) of a patient with haemorrhage. This is more clearly seen on the GE image due to magnetic susceptibility effects.

Mechanism

Magnetic susceptibility artefact occurs because all tissues magnetize to a different degree depending on their magnetic characteristics (see Chapter 1). This produces a difference in their individual precessional frequencies and phase. The phase discrepancy causes dephasing at the boundaries of structures with a very different magnetic susceptibility, and signal loss results.

Appearance

This artefact appears as areas of signal void and high signal intensity, often accompanied by distortion. It is commonly seen on gradient echo sequences when the patient has a metal prosthesis in situ as gradient rephasing cannot compensate for these magnetic field distortions (Figure 47.1). Magnetic susceptibility also occurs naturally such as at the interface of the petrous bone and the brain. Magnetic susceptibility can be used advantageously when investigating haemorrhage or blood products, as the presence of this artefact suggests that bleeding has recently occurred (Figure 47.2).

Remedy

• Using SE or FSE pulse sequences that use RF rephasing pulses (Figure 47.3).
• Removing all metal items from the patient before the examination.

axial abdomen slice, spins exhibit phase curve after phase-encoding gradient application

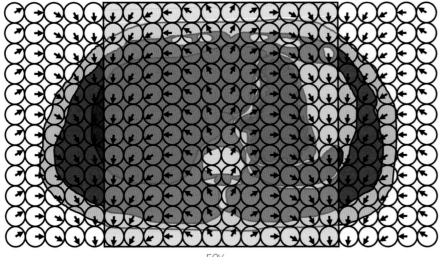

FOV

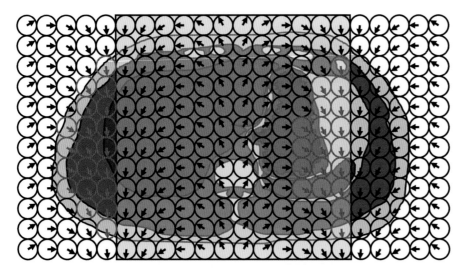

spins outside the field of view having same phase value as those inside

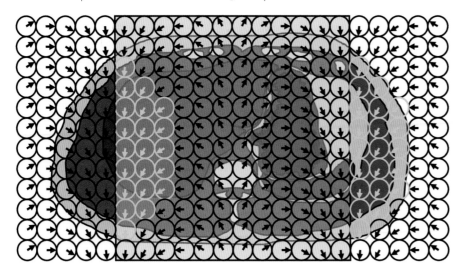

Figure 48.1 Aliasing or phase wrap.

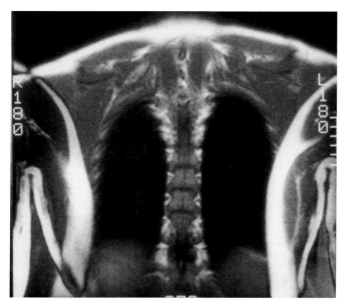

Figure 48.2 *Coronal image of the chest showing aliasing.*

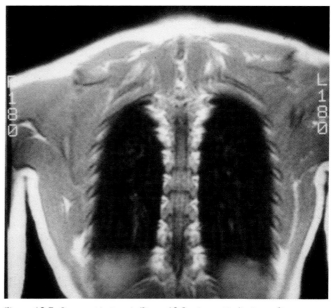

Figure 48.3 *Same patient as in Figure 48.2 using anti-aliasing software.*

Mechanism

Phase wrap/aliasing occurs when anatomy that is producing signal (as it is within the confines of the receiver coil) exists outside the FOV in the phase direction. Within the FOV, a finite number of phase values from 0° to 360° must be mapped into the FOV in the phase direction. This can be represented as a 'phase curve' that is repeated on either side of the FOV in the phase direction if anatomy, that is producing signal, exists here. Due to the finite number of phase values, signal coming outside the FOV has the same phase value as signal coming from inside, since they are both in the same position on the phase curve. There is therefore a duplication of phase values for anatomy inside and outside the FOV (Figure 48.1). It is caused by under-sampling of data when there is not enough data points in K space to accurately encode signal in the phase direction of the image.

Appearance

Anatomy outside the FOV in the phase direction is mapped onto the image. This is called **wrap around, fold-over** or **aliasing**. Anatomy from one side of the image overlaps the other (Figure 48.2). Severe forms can ruin an image.

Remedy

Aliasing can occur along the frequency axis but is usually automatically compensated for. Aliasing in the phase direction is reduced or eliminated in the following ways:

- Increasing the FOV to the boundaries of the coil.
- Placing spatial pre-saturation pulses over signal-producing anatomy.
- **Over-sampling** in the phase direction. This is specifically called **anti-aliasing**. During data acquisition the FOV is increased in the phase direction so that the phase curve now extends over twice the distance of the original FOV. There is now less likelihood of duplication of phase values of signal from anatomy outside the FOV although, to achieve this, more phase-encoding steps must be performed. This increases the scan time. On some systems the NEX/NSA maybe reduced to compensate for this. On these systems during image reconstruction the extra FOV is discarded (only the middle portion corresponding to the FOV selected is displayed). There is usually no penalty in scan time, signal or spatial resolution when using anti-aliasing on these systems, although motion artefact may be increased due to less signal averaging (see Chapter 39) (Figure 48.3).

49 Phase mismapping (motion artefact)

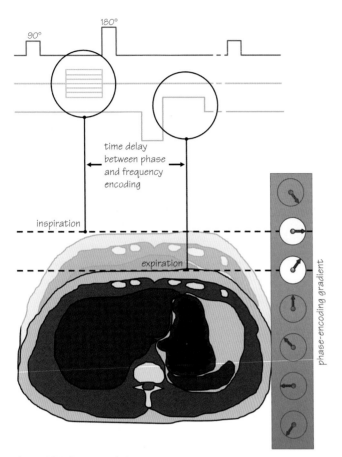

Figure 49.1 The cause of phase mismapping.

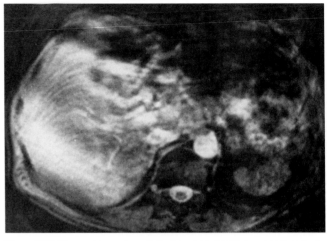

Figure 49.2 Phase mismapping artefact seen as ghosting across the image.

respiratory signal from bellows

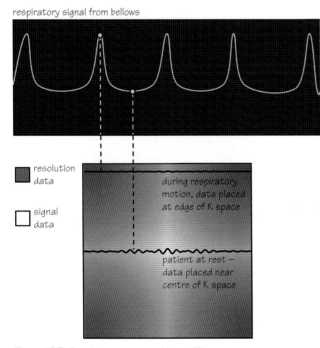

Figure 49.3 Respiratory compensation and K space.

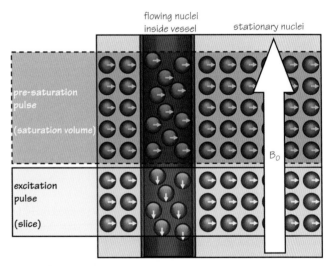

Figure 49.4 Spatial pre-saturation.

Mechanism

Phase artefact results from anatomy moving between the application of the phase-encoding gradient and the frequency-encoding gradient (intraview) and motion between each application of the phase gradient (view to view). If anatomy moves during these periods it is assigned the wrong phase value and is mismapped onto the image (Figure 49.1). It causes an artefact called **ghosting** or **phase mismapping** and always occurs along the phase axis of the image.

The most common causes of phase mismapping are respiration, which moves the chest and abdominal wall along the phase-encoding gradient, and pulsatile movement of artery or vein walls.

Appearance

Blurring or ghosting across the image (Figure 49.2).

Remedy

There are many ways of reducing phase mismapping. These are described below.

Respiratory compensation

Expandable air-filled **bellows** are placed around the patient's chest. The movement of air back and forth along the bellows during inspiration and expiration is converted to a waveform by a transducer. The system then orders the phase-encoding gradients so that the steep slopes occur when maximum movement of the chest wall occurs, and reserves the shallow gradient slopes (signal data) for minimum chest wall motion (Figure 49.3). In this way most of the signal is acquired when the chest wall is relatively still and therefore phase ghosting is reduced. Other techniques to reduce phase mismapping from respiratory motion include **breath-holding**, where the patient holds their breath during the acquisition of data, and **respiratory triggering** where data is only acquired when the chest wall is stationary.

Cardiac and peripheral gating

Cardiac and peripheral gating uses gating leads or sensors to obtain an ECG trace of the patient's cardiac activity. The system acquires data from each slice at the same phase of the cardiac cycle, thereby reducing phase mismapping from cardiac and vessel pulsation. Cardiac gating should be used when imaging the heart and great vessels. Peripheral gating is useful to reduce artefact from CSF flow.

Presaturation

Presaturation delivers a 90° RF pulse to a volume of tissue outside the FOV. This is called a **saturation band**. A flowing nucleus within the volume receives this 90° pulse. When it enters the slice stack, it receives an excitation pulse and is saturated. If it is fully saturated to 180°, it has no transverse component of magnetization and produces a signal void (Figure 49.4). To be effective, presaturation pulses should be placed between the flow and the imaging stack so that signal from flowing nuclei entering the FOV is nullified. Spatial saturation increases the rate of RF delivery to the patient; this increases the SAR.

Chemical presaturation

Chemical presaturation is used to produce a signal void in either fat or water. Hydrogen nuclei exist in two different chemical environments: The precessional frequencies of hydrogen in each environment are different. This precessional frequency shift is called **chemical shift** because it is caused by a difference in the chemical environments of fat and water. Chemical shift causes artefacts but also provides an opportunity to use a presaturation pulse to eliminate signal from either water or fat. This is called **chemical presaturation**.

• **Water Sat:** The chemical saturation RF pulse applied at the precessional frequency of water hydrogen shifts the NMV of water into saturation. The water hydrogen therefore has no transverse magnetization and thus no signal. When the signal from water is suppressed this is called **water suppression**.

• **Fat Sat:** The chemical saturation RF pulse is transmitted at the precessional frequency of fat hydrogen to shift the NMV of fat hydrogen into saturation. The fat hydrogen nuclei have no magnetization in the transverse plane and thus no signal. This is called **fat suppression**. There are various modifications to fat saturation that include adding gradient spoilers to spoil any transverse components of fat and using inversion sequences such as STIR (see Chapter 16).

Gradient moment rephasing

Gradient moment rephasing or **nulling/flow compensation** for the altered phase values of the nuclei flowing along a gradient (see Chapter 50) uses additional gradients to correct the altered phases back to their original values. In this way, flowing nuclei do not gain, or lose, phase due to the presence of the main gradient. Gradient moment rephasing therefore gives flowing nuclei a bright signal as they are in phase. As gradient moment rephasing uses extra gradients, it increases the minimum TE.

Increasing NSA/NEX

Increasing NSA/NEX reduces phase mismapping by averaging noise data. Phase mismapping is a form of noise and therefore, by averaging this data, its appearance in the image is reduced.

Note: Swapping the phase and frequency direction so that artefact is removed from the area of interest does **not** eliminate mismapping; it only moves it away from the area of interest and, as such, is not considered a technique that eliminates this artefact.

50 Flow phenomena

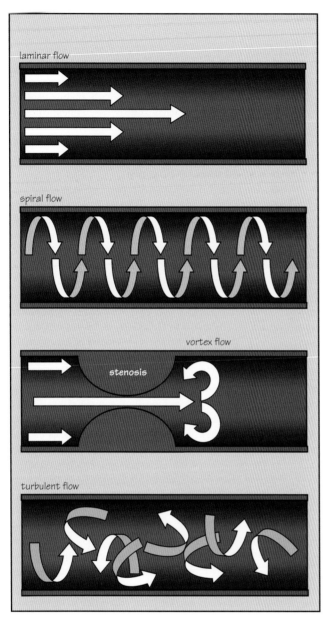

Figure 50.1 The different types of flow.

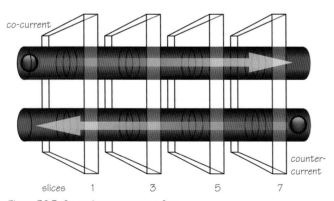

Figure 50.3 Co- and countercurrent flow.

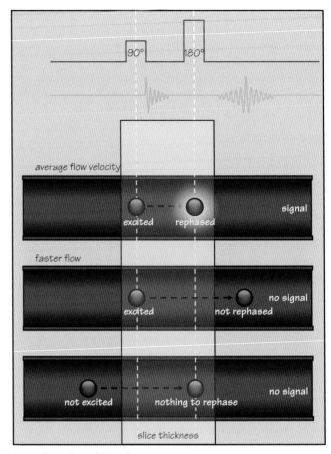

Figure 50.2 Time-of-flight flow phenomenon.

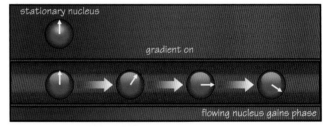

Figure 50.4 Intravoxel dephasing.

Laminar flow is flow that is at different but consistent velocities across a vessel. The flow at the centre of the lumen of the vessel is faster than at the vessel wall, where resistance slows down the flow. However, the velocity difference across the vessel is constant.

Turbulent flow is flow at different velocities that fluctuates randomly. The velocity difference across the vessel changes erratically.

Vortex flow is flow that is initially laminar but then passes through a stricture or stenosis in the vessel. Flow in the centre of the lumen has a high velocity, but near the walls the flow spirals.

Stagnant flow is where the velocity of flow slows to a point of stagnation. The signal intensity of stagnant flow depends on its T1, T2 and proton density characteristics. It behaves like stationary tissue (Figure 50.1).

- Only laminar flow can be compensated for.

Time-of-flight phenomenon

In order to produce a signal, a nucleus must receive an excitation pulse and a rephasing pulse. Stationary nuclei always receive both excitation and rephasing pulses. Flowing nuclei present in the slice for the excitation may have exited the slice before rephasing. This is called the **time-of-flight phenomenon**. If a nucleus receives the excitation pulse only and is not rephased, it does not produce a signal. If a nucleus is rephased but has not previously been excited, it does not produce a signal (Figure 50.2). Time-of-flight effects depend on:

- velocity of flow;
- TE;
- slice thickness.

Flow-related enhancement increases as:

- velocity of flow decreases;
- TE decreases;
- slice thickness increases.

High velocity signal loss increases as:

- velocity of flow increases;
- TE increases;
- slice thickness decreases.

Entry slice phenomenon (in-flow effect)

Entry slice phenomenon is related to the excitation history of the nuclei. Nuclei that receive repeated RF pulses during the acquisition are saturated. Nuclei that have not received these repeated RF pulses are 'fresh', as their magnetic moments have not been saturated by successive RF pulses. The signal that they produce is different to that of the saturated nuclei.

Stationary nuclei within a slice become saturated after repeated RF pulses. Nuclei flowing perpendicular to the slice enter the slice fresh, as they were not present during repeated excitations. They therefore produce a different signal to the stationary nuclei. This is called **entry slice phenomenon** as it is most prominent in the first slice of a 'stack' of slices. The slices in the middle of the stack exhibit less entry slice phenomenon, as flowing nuclei have received more excitation pulses by the time they reach these slices.

Any factor that affects the rate at which a nucleus receives repeated excitations affects the magnitude of the phenomenon. The magnitude of entry slice phenomenon therefore depends on:

- TR;
- slice thickness;
- velocity of flow;
- direction of flow.

Direction of flow

- **Co-current flow:** Flow that is in the **same** direction as slice selection is called **co-current**. The flowing nuclei are more likely to receive repeated RF excitations as they move from one slice to the next. They therefore become saturated relatively quickly, and so entry slice phenomenon decreases rapidly.
- **Countercurrent flow:** Flow that is in the **opposite** direction to slice selection is called **countercurrent** flow. Flowing nuclei stay fresh as when they enter a slice they are less likely to have received previous excitation pulses (Figure 50.3). Entry slice phenomenon does not therefore decrease rapidly and may still be present deep within the slice stack.

Intra-voxel dephasing

Nuclei flowing along a gradient rapidly accelerate or decelerate depending on the direction of flow and gradient application. Flowing nuclei either gain phase (if they have been accelerated), or lose phase (if they have been decelerated) (Figure 50.4). If a flowing nucleus is adjacent to a stationary nucleus in a voxel, there is a phase difference between the two nuclei. This is because the flowing nucleus has either lost or gained phase relative to the stationary nucleus due to its motion along the gradient. Nuclei within the same voxel are out of phase with each other, which results in a reduction of total signal amplitude from the voxel. This is called **intravoxel dephasing**.

51 Time-of-flight MR angiography

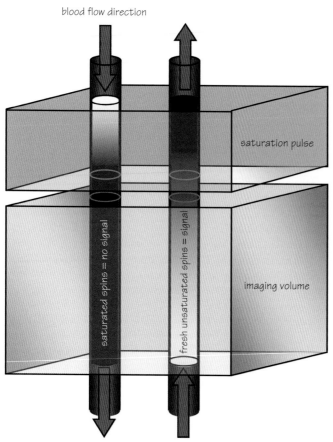

Figure 51.1 Presaturation volume relative to the imaging stack.

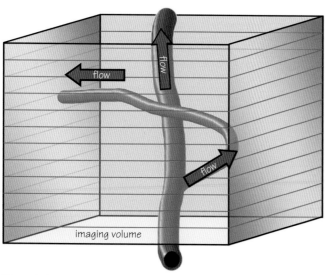

Figure 51.2 Flow and the imaging volume.

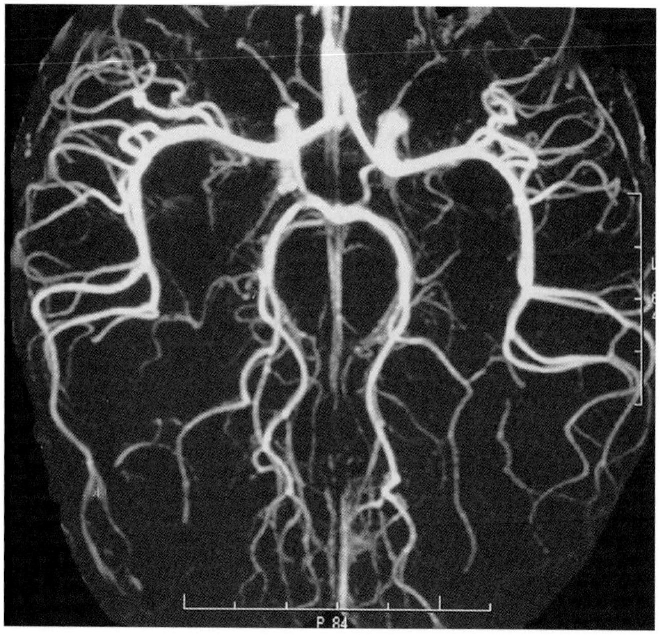

Figure 51.3 3D TOF MRA of a 4-year-old child showing normal appearances.

Mechanism

Time-of-flight MRA or **TOF MRA** produces vascular contrast by manipulating longitudinal magnetization of stationary spins. It uses a gradient echo pulse sequence in combination with GMN to enhance signal in flowing vessels. The TR is kept well below the T1 time of the stationary tissues so that T1 recovery is prevented. This saturates the stationary spins, while the inflow effect from fully magnetized flowing fresh spins produces high vascular signal. However, if the TR is too short, the flowing spins may be suppressed along with the stationary spins, and that has the effect of reducing vascular contrast. To evaluate signals from arterial flow, saturation pulses are applied in the direction of venous flow. For example, to evaluate the carotid arteries in the neck, apply saturation pulses superior to the imaging volume to saturate the signal from inflowing venous blood (Figure 51.1). TOF MRA is only sensitive to flow that comes into the FOV. Any flow that traverses the FOV can be saturated along with the stationary tissue (Figure 51.2).

2D vs 3D time-of-flight MRA

TOF MRA is acquired in either 2D (slice by slice) or 3D (volume) acquisition modes. In general, 3D volume imaging offers high SNR and thin contiguous slices for good resolution. However, as TOF MRA is sensitive to flow coming into the FOV or the imaging volume, spins in vessels with slow flow can be saturated in volume imaging. For this reason, 3D TOF should be used in areas of high velocity flow (intracranial applications), and 2D TOF in areas of slower velocity flow (carotids, peripheral vascular, and the venous systems). In 3D techniques, there is a higher risk of saturating signals from spins within the volume.

Clinical applications

The carotid bifurcation, the peripheral circulation and cortical venous mapping can be imaged with 2D TOF MRA (Figure 51.3).

Typical values

- **TR:** 45 ms
- **TE:** minimum allowable
- **Flip angle:** approx. 60°

- The TR and flip angle saturate stationary nuclei but moving spins coming into the slice remain fresh, so image contrast is maximized.
- The short TE reduces phase mismapping.
- Gradient moment rephasing, in conjunction with saturation pulses to suppress signals from areas of undesired flow, is used to enhance vascular contrast.

General advantages of TOF MRA

- Sensitive to T1 effects (short T1 tissues are bright; contrast may be given for additional enhancement).

- Reasonable imaging times (approximately 5 min depending on parameters).
- Sensitive to slow flow.
- Reduced sensitivity to intravoxel dephasing.

General disadvantages of TOF MRA

- Sensitive to T1 effects (short T1 tissues are bright so that haemorrhagic lesions may mimic vessels).
- Saturation of in-plane flow (any flow within the FOV or volume of tissue can be saturated along with background tissue).
- Enhancement is limited to either flow entering the FOV or very high velocity flow (Tables 51.1 and 51.2).

Table 51.1 Comparison of advantages and disadvantages of 2D and 3D time-of-flight MRA

Advantages of 2D TOF MRA	Disadvantages of 2D TOF MRA
Large area of coverage	Lower resolution
Sensitive to slow flow	Saturation of in-plane flow
Sensitive to T1 effects	Venetian blind artefact
Advantages of 3D TOF MRA	**Disadvantages of 3D TOF MRA**
High resolution for small vessels	Saturation of in-plane flow
Sensitive to T1 effects	Small area of coverage

Table 51.2 Overcoming disadvantages of time-of-flight MRA

Susceptibility artefacts	Use short TEs and small voxel volumes
Poor background suppression	Use TEs that acquire data when fat and water are out of phase
	Implement magnetization transfer techniques
Venetian blind artefacts	Use breath-hold techniques
Limited coverage (3D)	Acquire images in another plane
	Use MOTSA (multiple overlapping thin-section angiography)
Suppression of in-plane signal	Use ramped RF pulses
	Administer contrast media
Pulsation artefacts	Time acquisition to the cardiac cycle

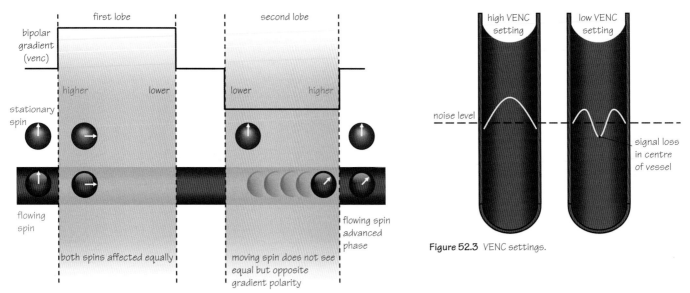

Figure 52.1 Bipolar gradients in phase contrast MRA.

Figure 52.3 VENC settings.

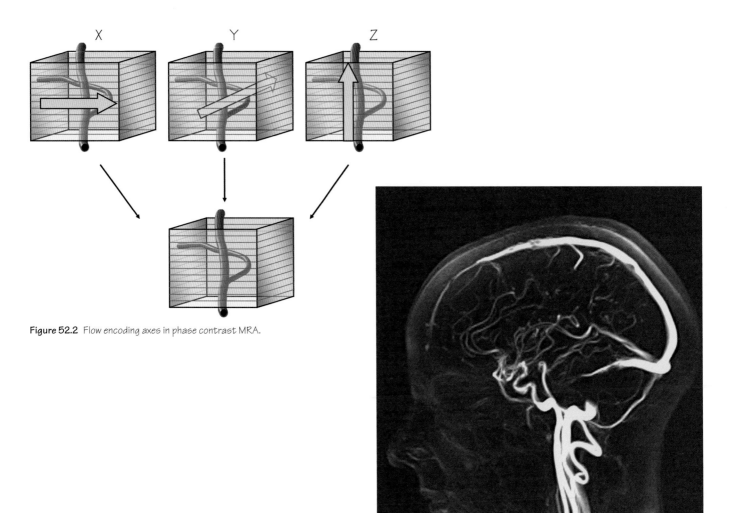

Figure 52.2 Flow encoding axes in phase contrast MRA.

Figure 52.4 PC venogram of the brain.

Mechanism

Phase contrast MRA utilizes velocity changes, and hence phase shifts in moving spins, to provide image contrast in flowing vessels. Phase shifts are generated in the pulse sequence by phase encoding the velocity of flow with the use of a bipolar (two lobes – one negative, one positive) gradient. Phase shift is introduced selectively for moving spins with the use of gradients. This technique is known as **phase contrast magnetic resonance angiography** or **PC MRA**. PC MRA is sensitive to flow within, as well as that coming into, the FOV.

• Immediately after the RF excitation pulse spins are in phase. A gradient is applied to both stationary and flowing spins. Although phase shifts occur in both stationary and flowing spins, these shifts occur at different rates.

• During initial application of the first bipolar gradient, there is a shift of phases of stationary spins and flowing spins.

• After the second part of the application of the first bipolar gradient, the stationary spins return to their initial phase, but those of moving spins acquire some phase (Figure 52.1).

• The bipolar gradient is then applied with opposite polarity so that the same variants occur, but in the opposite direction.

• PC MRA then subtracts the two acquisitions so that the signals from stationary spins are subtracted out, leaving only the signals from flowing spins. The combination of PC MRA acquisitions results in what are known as magnitude and phase images.

• The unsubtracted combinations of flow sensitized image data are known as **magnitude** images.

• The subtracted combinations are called **phase** images.

The bipolar gradients induce phase shifts along their axes. By applying bipolar gradients in all three axes the sequence is sensitized to flow in all three directions X, Y and Z. These are known as **flow encoding axes** (Figure 52.2). The sequence is also sensitized to flow velocity using a **velocity encoding technique** or **VENC** that compensates for projected flow velocity within vessels by controlling the amplitude or strength of the bipolar gradient. If the VENC selected is lower than the velocity within the vessel, aliasing can occur. This results in low signal intensity in the centre of the vessel, but better delineation of vessel wall itself. With high VENC settings, intraluminal signal is improved, but vessel wall delineation is compromised (Figure 52.3).

2D vs 3D phase contrast MRA (Table 52.1)

2D techniques provide acceptable imaging times and flow direction information. 2D acquisitions, however, cannot be reformatted and viewed in other imaging planes. 3D offers SNR and spatial resolution superior to 2D imaging strategies, and the ability to reformat in a number of imaging planes retrospectively. The trade-off, however, is that in 3D PC MRA, imaging time increases with the TR, NSA, the number of phase encoding steps, the number of slices and the number of flow encoding axes selected. For this reason, scan times are sometimes long.

Clinical uses

Phase contrast MRA can be used effectively in the evaluation of arteriovenous malformations, aneurysms, venous occlusions, congenital abnormalities and traumatic intracranial vascular injuries (Figure 52.4).

Typical values

3D volume acquisitions
• **Slices:** 28 slices volume, 1 mm slice thickness
• **Flip angle:** 20° (60-slice volume flip angle reduced to 15°)
• **TR:** ≤25 ms
• **VENC:** 40–60 cm/s
• **Flow encoding:** in all directions

2D techniques acquisitions
Cranial
• **TR:** 18–20 ms
• **Flip angle:** 20°
• **Slices:** thickness 20–60 mm
• **VENC:** 20–30 cm/s for venous flow
  40–60 cm/s for higher velocity with some aliasing
  60–80 cm/s to determine velocity and flow direction
Carotid
• **Flip angle:** 20–30°
• **TR:** 20 ms
• **VENC:** 40–60 cm/s for better morphology with aliasing
  60–80 cm/s for quantitative velocity and directional information

Table 52.1 Advantages and disadvantages of phase contrast MRA

Advantages	Disadvantages
Sensitivity to a variety of vascular velocities	Long imaging times with 3D
Sensitivity to flow within the FOV	More sensitive to turbulence
Reduced intra-voxel dephasing	
Increased background suppression	
Magnitude and phase images	

53 Contrast enhanced MR angiography

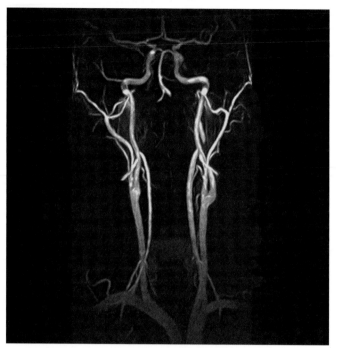

Figure 53.1 Coronal CE MRA of the carotid and vertebral arteries.

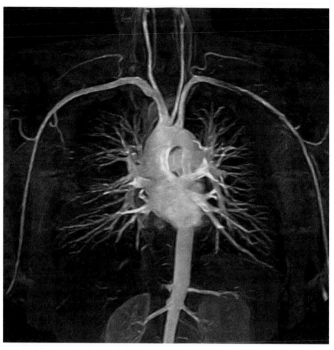

Figure 53.2 Coronal CE MRA of the chest.

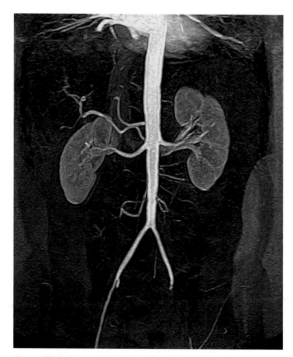

Figure 53.3 Coronal CE MRA of the abdominal vessels.

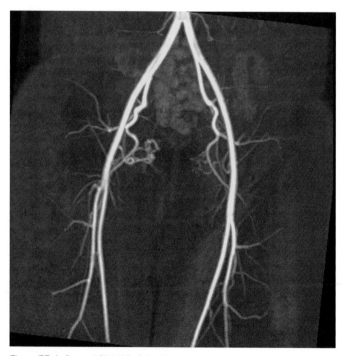

Figure 53.4 Coronal CE MRA of the iliac arteries showing an arteriovenous malformation.

Mechanism

Gadolinium is a T1 shortening agent that enhances blood if given in sufficient quantities into the bloodstream. If used in conjunction with a T1 weighted sequence, blood appears bright and is well seen in contrast to surrounding non-enhancing tissues (see Chapter 54) (Table 53.1, Figures 53.1, 53.2, 53.3 and 53.4). A conventional or fast incoherent gradient echo sequence should is used to keep scan times short.

Administration

Administration is intravenous, usually via the antecubital fossa by hand or mechanical injection.

Doses must be sufficiently high to give adequate visualization of vessels; 40–60 ml (about 0.3 mmol/kg) of gadolinium is required.

Image timing

To obtain an arterial-phase image in which arteries are bright and veins are dark, it is essential that the central K-space data (i.e. the low spatial frequency data) are acquired while gadolinium concentration in the arteries is high but relatively lower in the veins (see Chapter 39).

The time is it takes contrast to travel from the antecubital fossa to the area of interest depends on:

- distance of the area from the injection site;
- type of vessel (e.g. artery or vein);
- velocity of flow;
- speed of injection;
- length of the acquisition.

For long acquisitions, lasting more than 100 s, use sequential ordering of K space, so that the centre of K space is collected first (**centric K space filling**) (see Chapter 39). Sequential ordering results in fewer artefacts. Begin injecting the gadolinium just after initiating imaging. Finish the injection just after the midpoint of the acquisition, being careful to maintain the maximum injection rate for the approximately 10–30 s prior to the middle of the acquisition. This will ensure a maximum arterial gadolinium during the middle of the acquisition when central K-space data are collected.

For short acquisitions, less than 45 s contrast agent bolus timing is more critical and challenging. There are several approaches to determining the optimal bolus timing for these fast scans. For a typical breath-hold scan duration of 35–45 s in a reasonably healthy patient with an intravenous site in the antecubital vein, a delay of approximately 10–12 s is appropriate. Therefore, begin the injection, and then 10 s later start imaging while the patient suspends breathing.

More reliable and precise techniques are also available. These include:
- using a test bolus to precisely measure the contrast travel time;
- using an automatic pulse sequence that monitors signal in the aorta and then initiates imaging after contrast is detected arriving in the aorta;
- imaging so rapidly that bolus timing is unimportant.

Table 53.1 Advantages and disadvantages of contrast enhanced MRA

Advantages	Disadvantages
Easier to visualize vessels – fewer false positives	Timing is sometimes difficult
No extra sequences needed	Invasive – risk of reaction
With practice examination complete in 15–30 mins	Extra equipment such as power injectors and moving tables may be required

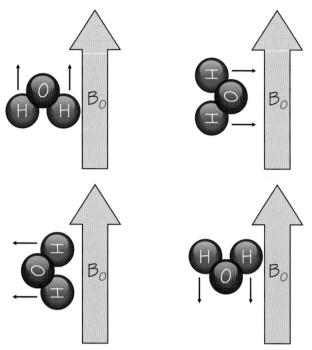

Figure 54.1 Tumbling of water molecules.

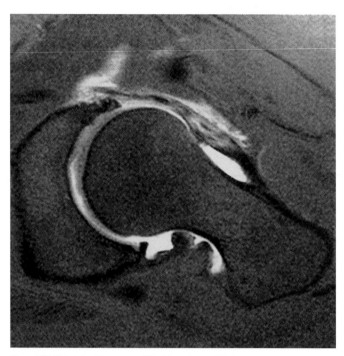

Figure 54.2 Axial arthrogram of the hip using gadolinium.

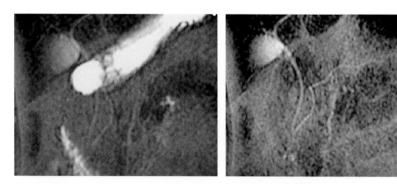

Figure 54.3 Biliary system before (left) and after (right) oral iron oxide agent.

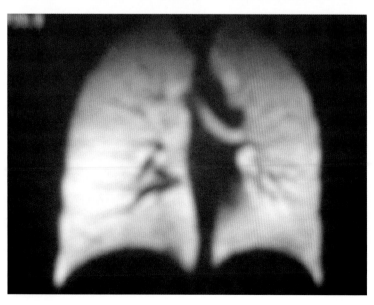

Figure 54.4 Lungs after inhalation of hyper-polarized helium.

Mechanism

In order to increase contrast between pathology and normal tissue, enhancement agents may be introduced that selectively affect the T1 and T2 relaxation times in tissues. Both T1 recovery and T2 decay are influenced by the magnetic field experienced locally within the nucleus. The local magnetic field responsible for these processes is caused by:
- the main magnetic field;
- fluctuations caused by the magnetic moments of nuclear spins in neighbouring molecules.

These molecules rotate or tumble, and the rate of rotation of the molecules is a characteristic property of the solution. It is dependent on:
- magnetic field strength;
- viscosity of the solution;
- temperature of the solution.

Molecules that tumble with a frequency at or near the Larmor frequency have more efficient T1 recovery times than other molecules (Figure 54.1).

Dipole-dipole interactions

The phenomenon by which excited protons are affected by nearby excited protons and electrons is called **dipole-dipole** interaction. If a tumbling molecule with a large magnetic moment such as gadolinium is placed in the presence of water protons, local magnetic field fluctuations occur near the Larmor frequency. T1 relaxation times of nearby protons are therefore reduced and so they appear bright on a T1 weighted image. This effect on a substance whereby relaxation rates are altered is known as **relaxivity**.

Gadolinium

Gadolinium (Gd) is a **paramagnetic** agent. It is a trivalent lanthanide element that has seven unpaired electrons and an ability to allow rapid exchange of bulk water to minimize the space between itself and water within the body. It has a large magnetic moment and, when it is placed in the presence of tumbling water protons, fluctuations in the local magnetic field are created near the Larmor frequency. The T1 relaxation times of nearby water protons are therefore reduced, resulting in an increased signal intensity on T1 weighted images. For this reason, gadolinium is known as a **T1 enhancement agent**.

Chelation

Gadolinium is a rare earth metal that cannot be excreted by the body and would cause long-term side effects as it binds to membranes. By binding the gadolinium ion to a **chelate** such as diethylene triaminepentaacetic acid (DTPA) (a ligand), the chelate compound Gd-DTPA is formed which can be safely excreted. Other chelate compounds include:
- Gd-HP-DO3A in which the charges have been balanced to produce a non-ionic contrast agent;
- Gd-DTPA-BMA (gadodiamide), a non-ionic linear molecule;
- Gd-DOTA, an ionic macrocyclic molecule.

Side effects

- A slight transitory increase in bilirubin and blood iron.
- Mild transitory headaches.
- Nausea.
- Vomiting.
- Hypotension.
- Gastrointestinal upset.
- Rash.

Contra-indications

- Haematological disorders such as haemolytic anaemia.
- Sickle cell anaemia.
- Pregnancy.

Administration

The effective dosage of Gd-DTPA is 0.1 millimoles per kilogram of body weight (mmol/kg) (approx. 0.2 ml/kg or 0.1 ml/lb.), with a maximum dose of 20 ml. Gd-HP-DO3A has been approved for up to 0.3 mmol/kg or three times the dose of Gd-DTPA.

Clinical applications

Gadolinium has proven invaluable in imaging the central nervous system because of its ability to pass through breakdowns in the blood–brain barrier (BBB). Clinical indications for gadolinium include:
- tumours;
- infection;
- arthrography (Figure 54.2);
- post-operation lumbar disc;
- breast disease;
- vessel patency and morphology (see Chapter 53).

Iron oxide

Iron oxides shorten relaxation times of nearby hydrogen atoms and therefore reduce the signal intensity in normal tissues. This results in a signal loss on proton density weighted or heavily T2 weighted images. Superparamagnetic iron oxides are known as **T2 enhancement agents**. Iron oxide is taken up by the reticuloendothelial system and excreted by the liver so that normal liver is dark and liver lesions are bright on T2 weighted images.

Side effects

- Mild to severe back, leg and groin pain.
- Nausea, vomiting and diarrhoea.
- Anaphylactic-like reactions.

Contraindications

Iron oxide is contraindicated in patients with known allergies or hypersensitivity to iron, parenteral dextran, parenteral iron-dextran or parenteral iron polysaccharide preparations.

Administration

The recommended dose of iron oxide is 0.56 mg of iron per kg of body weight. This should be diluted in 100 ml of 50% dextrose and given intravenously over 30 min. The diluted drug is administered through a 5-micron filter at a rate of 2–4 mmol/min. This agent should be used within 8 hours following dilution.

Clinical applications

Iron oxide is mainly used in liver and biliary imaging (Figure 54.3).

Other contrast agents

Gastrointestinal contrast agents are sometimes used for bowel enhancement. Theses include barium, ferromagnetic agents and fatty substances. However, due to constant peristalsis, these agents enhance bowel motion artefacts more often than enhancing pathological lesions. The use of antispasmodic agents helps to retard peristalsis to decrease these artefacts. Other agents include helium that is inhaled and assists in the evaluation of lung perfusion (Figure 54.4).

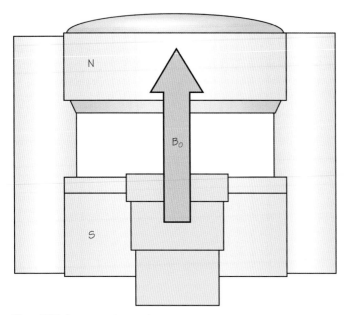

Figure 55.1 A permanent magnet.

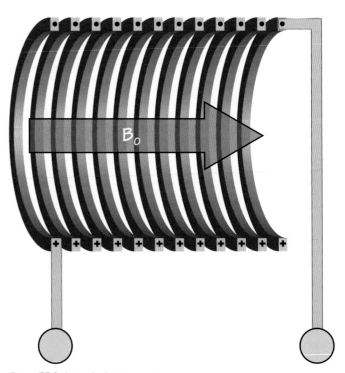

Figure 55.2 A simple electromagnet.

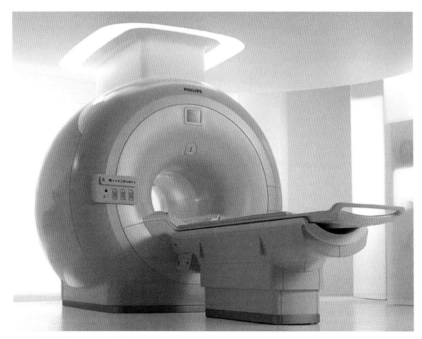

Figure 55.3 A superconducting system.

Permanent magnets

Permanent magnets consist of ferromagnetic substances which have magnetic susceptibility greater than 1. They are easily magnetized and retain this magnetization (Figure 55.1). Examples of substances used are iron, cobalt, and nickel. The most common material used is an alloy of aluminium, nickel and cobalt, known as **alnico**.

Advantages

• Open design: children, obese and claustrophobic patients scanned with ease. Interventional and dynamic procedures possible.
• They require no power supply, and operating costs are therefore low.
• The magnetic field created by a permanent magnet has lines of flux running vertically, keeping the magnetic field virtually confined within the boundaries of the scan room.

Disadvantages

• Excessive weight, only low fixed field-strengths (0.2–0.3 T) can be achieved.
• Longer scan times due to lower field strengths.

Electromagnets

Electromagnets utilize the laws of electromagnetic induction by passing an electrical current through a series of wires to produce a magnetic field (see Chapter 1). This physical phenomenon is utilized to produce RF coils and the static magnetic field.

Resistive magnets

The magnetic field strength in a resistive magnet is dependent on the current which passes through its coils of wire. The direction of the main magnetic field in a resistive magnet follows the right-hand thumb rule and produces lines of flux running horizontally from the head to the foot of the magnet (see Chapter 1) (Figure 55.2).

Advantages

• Lighter in weight than the permanent magnet.
• Capital costs are low.

Disadvantages

• The operational costs of the resistive magnet are quite high due to the large quantities of power required to maintain the magnetic field.
• The maximum field strength in an system of this type is less than 0.3 T due to its excessive power requirements. Therefore scan times are longer.
• The resistive system is relatively safe as the field can be turned off instantaneously. However, this type of magnet does create significant stray fringe magnetic fields.

Superconducting electromagnets

The resistance of the coils of wire is dependent on the material of which the loops of wire are made, the length of the wire in the loop, the cross-sectional area of the wire, and temperature. The latter can be controlled so that resistance is minimized.

As resistance decreases, the current dissipation also decreases. Therefore if the resistance is reduced, the energy required to maintain the magnetic field is decreased. As temperature decreases, resistance also decreases. As absolute zero of temperature ($-273°$C or $4°$K) is approached resistance is virtually absent, so that a high magnetic field can be maintained with no input power or driving voltage required. This is the basis of the function of the supercooled, superconducting magnet. The direction of the main magnetic field runs horizontally like that of the resistive system, from the head to the feet of the magnet.

Initially, current is passed through the loops of wire to create the magnetic field or bring the field up to strength (ramping). Then the wires are supercooled with substances known as cryogens (usually liquid helium [He] or liquid nitrogen [N]), to eliminate resistance. Since He and N are stable, they can be placed into a vacuum so that they do not rapidly boil off or return to their gaseous state. This is called a **cryogen bath** that actually surrounds the coils of wire and is housed in the system between insulated vacuums (Figure 55.3).

Advantages

• High magnetic field strengths with low power requirements (after the magnetic field has been ramped up) (0.5–12 T).
• Low operating cost. With resistance virtually eliminated, there is no longer a mechanism to dissipate current, therefore no additional power input is required to maintain the high magnetic field strength.
• Advanced applications and optimum image quality.

Disadvantages

• High capital cost.
• Fringe fields are significant so shielding is necessary.
• Tunnel design renders it unsuitable for large or claustrophobic patients. Interventional and dynamic studies are also difficult.

Shim coils

Due to design limitations it is almost impossible to create an electromagnet with coils of wire that are spaced evenly (equidistant from one end of the solenoid to the other). As the strength of the field is dependent on the distance between the loops, unevenly spaced loops create sags or **inhomogeneities** in the main magnetic field. These are measured in parts per million (ppm).

To correct for these inhomogeneities, another loop of current-carrying wire is placed in the area of the inhomogeneity. This, in effect, compensates for the sag in the main magnetic field and thus creates magnetic field homogeneity or evenness. This process is called **shimming** and the extra loop of wire is called a **shim** coil. For imaging purposes, homogeneity on the order of 10 ppm is required. Spectroscopic procedures require a more homogeneous environment of 1 ppm.

56 Gradients

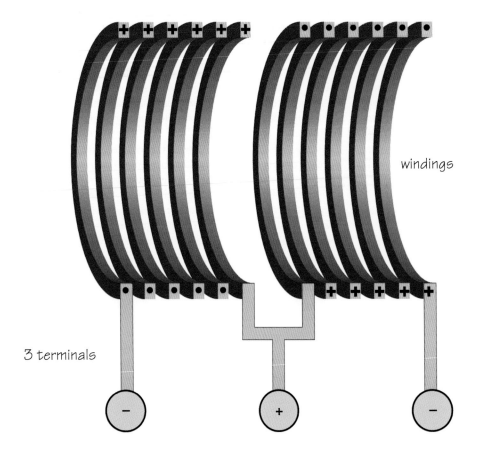

3 terminals

windings

Figure 56.1 A three-terminal electromagnet used in gradient coils.

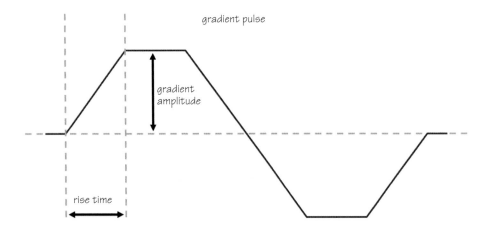

gradient pulse

gradient amplitude

rise time

Figure 56.2 Gradient amplitude and rise time.

Gradient coils provide a linear gradation or slope of the magnetic field strength from one end of the magnet to the other. This is achieved by passing current through the gradient coils (see Chapter 27).

• The direction of the current through the coil determines whether the magnetic field strength is increased or decreased relative to isocentre, i.e. its polarity.

• The polarity of the current flowing through the coil determines which end of the gradient is higher than isocentre (positive) and which end is lower (negative) (Figure 56.1).

Gradient coils are powered by **gradient amplifiers**. There are two gradient amplifiers for each gradient, one affixed to the high end of the gradient, the other to the low. Faults in the gradients or gradient amplifiers can result in geometric distortions in the MR image.

By varying the magnetic field strength, gradients provide position-dependent variation of signal frequency and are therefore used for:

• slice selection;
• frequency encoding;
• phase encoding;
• rewinding;
• spoiling.

To apply a gradient, current is passed through a gradient coil. The change in field strength gradually increases to maximum dependent on the magnitude of the current. The gradient remains at maximum for a specific period of time and is then switched off. The change in field strength gradually decreases until there is no change, i.e. the magnetic field strength along the bore is equal to the main field strength of the magnet.

The **maximum amplitude** of a gradient is the maximum change of field strength per metre along the bore of the magnet that is achievable. This factor determines the maximum resolution possible because:

• Steep slice select gradients are required for thin slices.
• Steep phase-encoding gradients are required for fine phase matrices.
• Steep frequency-encoding gradients are required for small fields of view.

• The **rise time** of a gradient is the time required to achieve the maximum amplitude.

• The **slew rate** is a function of rise time and amplitude. These factors determine the shortest scan times achievable.

• The **duty cycle** is the percentage of time the gradient is at maximum amplitude (Figure 56.2).

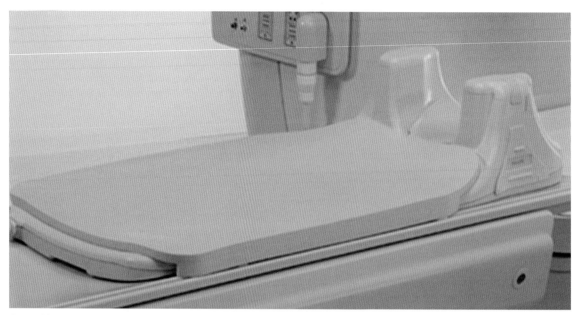

Figure 57.1 Spinal phased array coil.

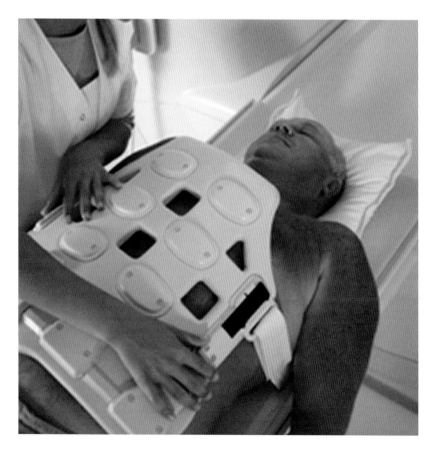

Figure 57.2 Parallel imaging coils.

RF coils consist of loops of wire which, when a current is passed through them, produce a magnetic field at 90° to B_0.

Transmit coils

Energy is transmitted at the resonant frequency of hydrogen in the form of a short intense burst of radiofrequency known as a radiofrequency pulse.

The main coils that transmit RF in most systems are:
- a body coil usually located within the bore of the magnet;
- a head coil.

The body coil is the main RF transmitter and transmits RF for most examinations excluding head imaging (when the head coil is used). The body and head coil are also capable of receiving RF, i.e. acting as receiver coils.

Receiver coils

RF coils placed in the transverse plane generate a voltage when a moving magnetic field cuts across the loops of wire. This voltage is the MR signal that is sampled to form an image. In order to induce an MR signal, the transverse magnetization must occur perpendicular to the receiver coils.

RF coil types

The configuration of the RF transmitter and receiver coils directly affects the quality of the MR signal. There are several types of coil currently used in MR imaging.

Transmit/Receive coils

A coil both transmits RF and receives the MR signal and is often called a **transceiver**. It encompasses the entire anatomy and can be used for either head or total body imaging. Head and body coils of a type known as the birdcage configuration are used to image relatively large areas and yield uniform SNR over the entire imaging volume. However, even though the volume coils are responsible for uniform excitation over a large area, because of their large size they generally produce images with lower SNR than other types of coil. The signal quality produced by these coils has been significantly increased by a process known as **quadrature excitation and detection**.

Surface coils

Coils of this type are used to improve the SNR when imaging structures near the surface of the patient. Generally, the nearer the coil is situated to the structure under examination, the greater the SNR. This is because the coil is closer to the signal-emitting anatomy, and only noise in the vicinity of the coil is received rather than the entire body.

Surface coils are usually small and especially shaped so that they can be easily placed near the anatomy to be imaged with little or no discomfort to the patient. However, signal (and noise) is received only from the sensitive volume of the coil which corresponds to the area located around the coil. The size of this area extends to the circumference of the coil and at a depth into the patient equal to the radius of the coil. There is therefore a fall-off of signal as the distance from the coil is increased in any direction.

Intracavity coils (such as rectal coils) or local coils can be used to receive signal deep within the patient. As the SNR is enhanced when using local coils, greater spatial resolution of small structures can often be achieved. When using local coils, the body coil is used to transmit RF and the local coil is used to receive the MR signal.

Phased array coils

These consist of multiple coils and receivers whose individual signals are combined to create one image with improved SNR and increased coverage. Therefore the advantages of small surface coils (increased SNR and resolution) are combined with a large FOV for increased anatomy coverage. Usually up to four coils and receivers are grouped together to either increase longitudinal coverage or to improve uniformity across a whole volume. During data acquisition, each individual coil receives signal from its own small usable FOV. The signal output from each coil is separately received and processed but then combined to form one single, larger FOV. As each coil has its own receiver, the amount of noise received is limited to its small FOV, and all the data are acquired in a single sequence rather than in four individual sequences (Figure 57.1).

Parallel imaging coils

Parallel imaging technology has been discussed previously (see Chapter 39). This technique uses multiple coils (also known as channels) placed around the imaging volume (Figure 57.2). During each acquisition each coil sends data to its own unique K-space line so that K space is filled more rapidly. For example, if four coils or channels are used, K space may be filled four lines at a time. This technique can be used with any sequence.

Large coil
- Large area of uniform signal reception.
- Increased likelihood of aliasing with small FOV.
- Positioning of patient not too critical.
- Lower SNR and resolution.

Small coil
- Small area of signal reception.
- Less likely to produce aliasing artefact.
- Positioning of coil critical.
- High SNR and resolution.

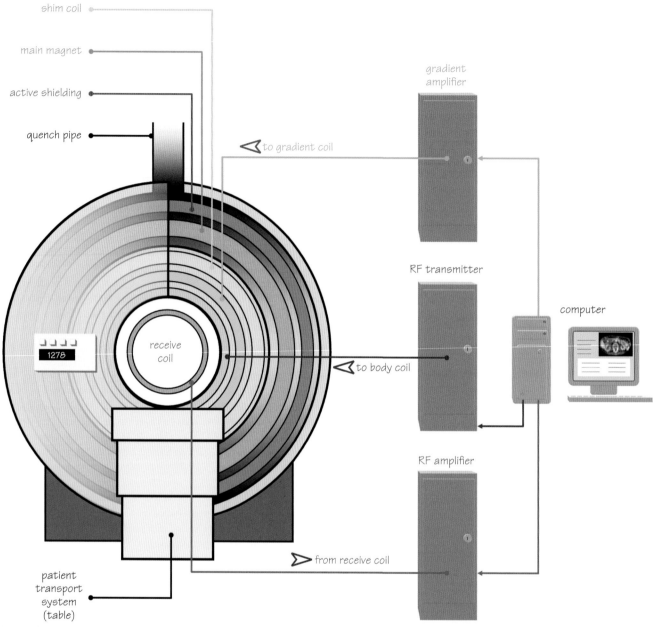

Figure 58.1 MR instrumentation.

The pulse control unit

The pulse control unit is responsible for synchronizing the application of the gradients and RF pulses in a pulse sequence.

• Gradient coils are switched on and off very rapidly and at precise times during the pulse sequence.

• Gradient amplifiers supply the power to the gradient coils and a pulse control unit coordinates the functions of the gradient amplifiers and the coils so that they can be switched on and off at the appropriate times.

• RF at the resonant frequency is transmitted by the RF transceiver, passes through frequency synthesizers to the RF amplifier and then through an RF monitor which ensures that safe levels of RF are delivered to the patient.

• The received RF signal from the coil is filtered, amplified and digitized and then passes to the array processor for fast Fourier transform (FFT). This data is then transmitted to the image processor so that each pixel can be allocated a grey scale colour in the image (Figure 58.1).

The operator interface

MRI computer systems vary with manufacturer. Most consist of:

• a minicomputer with expansion capabilities;

• an array processor for Fourier transformation;

• an image processor that takes data from the array processor to form an image;

• hard disc drives for storage of raw data and pulse sequence parameters;

• a power distribution mechanism to distribute and filter the alternating current.

Data storage

For permanent storage of MR image data, data may be archived to an optical disc. Images are stored for viewing by a radiologist and so that cases can be retrieved for further manipulation and imaging in the future. They may also be used for comparison when repeat examinations are performed on the same patient.

59 Bioeffects

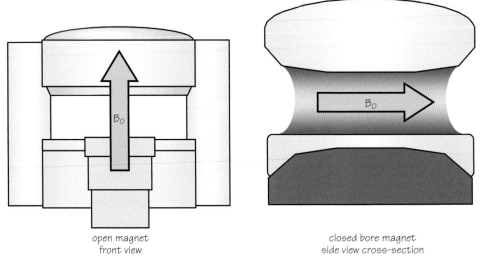

open magnet
front view

closed bore magnet
side view cross-section

Figure 59.1 Static field in permanent and superconducting systems.

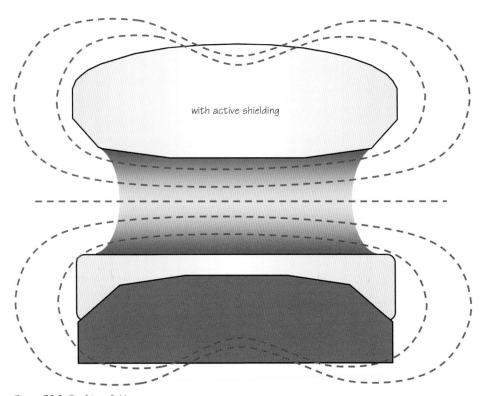

with active shielding

Figure 59.2 The fringe field.

Static magnetic field bioeffects

Current guidelines recommend a maximum limit of 8 T for clinical imaging rising to 12 T for research purposes and spectroscopy. Most clinical units operate below 3 T.

The following points are *fundamentally* important with regard to the potentially harmful effects of the static magnetic field:
- The static field is always present (24 hours a day, 365 days a year to infinity). It is switched on even when the system is out of use (Figure 59.1).
- The fringe field may extend several meters beyond the examination room and therefore any harmful effects or risks may come into play at some distance from the scanner (Figure 59.2).

There is no conclusive evidence for irreversible or harmful bioeffects in humans below 2.5 T. Reversible abnormalities may include:
- an increase in the amplitude of the T-wave can be noted on an ECG due to the magnetic hydrodynamic effect (also known as the magnetic haemodynamic effect);
- heating of patients;
- fatigue;
- headaches;
- hypotension;
- irritability.

Time-varying field bioeffects

Gradients create a time-varying magnetic field. This changing field occurs during the scanning sequence. It is not present at other times and therefore exposure is restricted to patients and to relatives who may be present in the scan room during the examination.

The health consequences are not related to the strength of the gradient field, but to changes in the magnetic field that cause induced currents. Nerves, blood vessels and muscles, which act as conductors in the body, may be affected. The induced current is greater in peripheral tissues since the amplitude of the gradient is higher away from magnetic isocentre.

Time-varying bioeffects from gradient coils include:
- light flashes in the eyes;
- alterations in the biochemistry of cells and fracture union;
- mild cutaneous sensations;
- involuntary muscle contractions;
- cardiac arrhythmias.

RF transmit coils also produce time-varying fields. The predominant biological effect of RF irradiation absorption is the potential heating of tissue. As an excitation pulse is applied, some nuclei absorb the RF energy and enter the high-energy state. As they relax, nuclei give off this absorbed energy to the surrounding lattice. As excitation frequency is increased, absorbed energy is also increased, therefore heating of tissue is largely frequency dependent.

Energy dissipation can be described in terms of **specific absorption rate** or **SAR**. SAR is expressed in watts per kilogram (W/kg), a quantity that depends on:
- induced electric field;
- pulse duty cycle;
- tissue density;
- conductivity;
- the size of the patient.

SAR is used to calculate an expected increase in body temperature, during an average examination. In the UK, it is recommended that this should not exceed 1°C during the examination.

Studies show that patient exposure up to three times the recommended levels produces no serious adverse effects, despite elevations in skin and body temperatures. As body temperature increases, blood pressure and heart rate also increase slightly. Even though these effects seem insignificant, patients with compromised thermoregulatory systems may not be candidates for MR.

Radio frequency fields can be responsible for significant burn hazards due to electrical currents that are produced in conductive loops. Equipment used in MRI, such as ECG leads and surface coils, should therefore be used with extreme caution. When using a surface coil, the operator must be careful to prevent any electrically conductive material (e.g. cable of surface coil) from forming a 'conductive loop' with itself or with the patient.

60 Projectiles

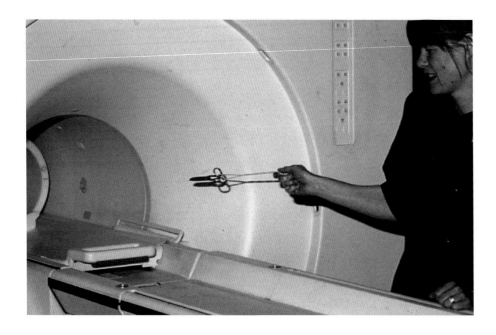

Figure 60.1 The pulling power of a pair of scissors in a 1.5 T system.

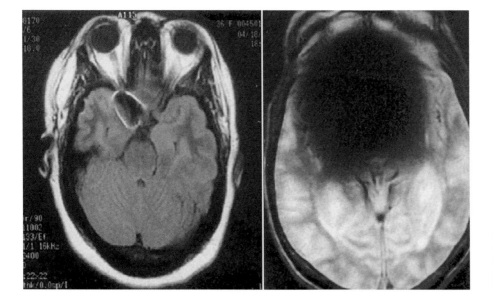

Figure 60.2 Patient with an intracranial vascular clip using spin echo (left) and gradient echo MRI (right). Magnetic susceptibility artefact is clearly seen on the gradient echo image.

The projectile effect of a metal object exposed to the field can seriously compromise the safety of anyone sited between the object and the magnet system. **The potential harm cannot be overemphasized.** Even small objects such as paperclips and hairpins have a terminal velocity of 40 mph when pulled into a 1.5 T magnet, and therefore pose a serious risk to the patient and anyone else present in the scan room. Larger objects such as scissors travel at much higher velocities and may be fatal to any person in its path (Figure 60.1).

Many types of clinical equipment are ferromagnetic and should **never** be brought into the scan room. These include:

- surgical tools;
- scissors;
- clamps;
- oxygen tanks.

Metallic implants and prostheses

Metallic implants and prostheses produce serious effects which include torque or twisting in the field, heating effects and artefacts on MR images. The type of metal used in such implants is one factor that determines the force exerted on them in magnetic fields. While non-ferrous metallic implants may show little or no deflection to the field, they could cause significant heating due to their inability to dissipate the heat caused by radiofrequency absorption.

Intracranial aneurysm clips

Clip motion may damage the vessel, resulting in haemorrhage, ischaemia or death. Currently, many intracranial clips are made of a non-ferromagnetic substance such as titanium. However, recent studies have indicated that even these may deflect in a magnetic field. It is therefore recommended that imaging of patients with aneurysm clips is delayed, until the type of clip is emphatically identified as non-ferrous and non-deflectable. Intracranial clips also cause severe magnetic susceptibility artefact, especially in gradient echo sequences (Figure 60.2).

Cardiac pacemakers

Even field strengths as low as 10 gauss may be sufficient to cause deflection, programming changes, and closure of the reed switch that converts a pacemaker to asynchronous mode. In addition, patients who have had their pacemaker removed may have pacer wires left within the body that could act as an antenna and (by induced currents) cause cardiac fibrillation.

Prosthetic heart valves

Prosthetic heart valves are considerably deflected by the static magnetic field. The deflection, however, is minimal compared to normal pulsatile cardiac motion. Therefore, although patients with most valvular implants are considered safe for MR, as there are valves whose integrity is compromised, careful screening for valve type is advised.

Cochlear implants

Cochlear implants are attracted to the magnetic field and are magnetically or electronically activated.

Intraocular ferrous foreign bodies

It is not uncommon for patients who have worked with sheet metal to have metal fragments or slivers located in and around the eye. Since the magnetic field exerts a force on ferromagnetic objects, a metal fragment in the eye could move or be displaced and cause injury to the eye or surrounding tissue. Therefore all patients with a suspected eye injury must be X-rayed before the MR examination.

Orthopaedic implants

Most orthopaedic implants show no deflection within the main magnetic field. A large metallic implant such as a hip prosthesis can become heated by currents induced in the metal by the magnetic and radiofrequency fields. It appears, however, that such heating is relatively low. The majority of orthopaedic implants have been imaged with MR without incident.

Abdominal surgical clips

Abdominal surgical clips are generally safe for MR because they become anchored by fibrous tissue, but produce artefacts in proportion to their size and can distort the image.

61 Screening and safety procedures

Due to the hazards particularly associated with projectiles, all persons entering the controlled area must satisfy a safety screening procedure. In addition, it is advised that all nursing, housekeeping, fire department, emergency and MR personnel are educated about the potential risks and hazards of the static magnetic field. Signs should be attached at all entrances to the magnetic field (including the fringe field), to deter entry into the scan room with ferromagnetic objects.

Screening procedure
Two distinct safety zones may be identified around the MR system.

The exclusion zone
The exclusion zone is defined by the boundary of the 5 gauss line. A warning sign should be posted at all points of access to the exclusion zone. Entrance must be restricted to those people who have passed the screening procedure. In modern scanners the 5 G line is usually within the exclusion zone.

The security zone
The security zone is an area, usually the magnet room itself, where the potential to cause projectile injuries exists due to the attraction of loose objects into the magnet.

Security zone precautions
• Have only one point of access, marked by a warning sign. People entering the scan room must be screened for any loose ferromagnetic objects prior to entry.
• The scan room door should be kept closed at all times when not in use.
• Patients must not be left unattended within the magnet room.

Several measures must be taken to ensure that no person approaches the magnetic field that could pose a risk to either themselves or patients.
• There must be at least two physical barriers between the 5 G line and general public access. Lockable or magnetically switched doors and gates are preferable. Every barrier must clearly display a sign warning of the presence of a strong magnetic field, with a list of devices that must not enter beyond this point (e.g. pacemakers). These barriers and signs must be displayed 24 hours a day.
• There must be thorough screening of *every* person who is to enter the field, including radiographers, doctors, patients, relatives, cleaners and porters. There are no exceptions.

All centres should have a proper screening policy that includes checking for:
• pacemakers;
• intraocular foreign bodies;
• metal devices or prostheses;
• cochlear implants;
• possibility of early pregnancy.

Most facilities provide a screening form that patients, relatives and other persons fill in before entering the magnetic field. This ensures that important questions have been addressed, and provides a record that screening has taken place. This may be critical if an accident subsequently occurs.

Items such as watches, credit cards, money, pens and any other loose items must be removed before entering the magnetic field. Unremovable items such as splints must be thoroughly checked for safety with a hand-held bar magnet before entering the MR scan room.

Staff safety
Permanent personnel such as radiographers, radiologists and clerical staff need only complete a safety questionnaire at their first visit to the unit. Other staff such as visiting doctors or nurses accompanying patients must complete a safety form and remove all loose items at each visit if they are entering the magnetic field.

Exposure to gradient and radiofrequency fields only occurs during the scan sequence and therefore staff are not usually subjected to it. However there are occasions when staff are required to be present in the room during the sequence.

While a patient is only exposed to these fields for the short duration of the examination, staff under these circumstances may be subjected to repeated exposures. At present some exposure to changing fields on an occasional basis is not thought to be harmful.

Pregnancy
As yet, there are no known biological effects of MRI on fetuses. However, there are a number of mechanisms that could potentially cause adverse effects as a result of the interaction of electromagnetic fields with developing fetuses. Cells undergoing division, which occurs during the first trimester of pregnancy, are more susceptible to these effects.

Any examination of pregnant patients should be delayed until the end of the first trimester and then a written consent form should be signed by the patient before the examination. However, if the patient has a life-threatening illness and the only alternative imaging involves ionizing radiation, MRI should be considered.

MR facilities have established individual guidelines for pregnant employees in the magnetic resonance environment. The majority of units have determined that pregnant employees can safely enter the scan room, but should leave while the RF and gradient fields are employed. Some facilities, however, recommend that the employee stay out of the magnetic field entirely during the first trimester of pregnancy.

Emergencies in the MR environment

Quenching

Quenching is the process whereby there is a sudden loss of absolute zero of temperature in the magnet coils, so that they cease to be superconducting and become resistive. This results in helium escaping from the cryogen bath extremely rapidly. It may happen accidentally or can be manually instigated in the case of an emergency. Quenching may cause severe and irreparable damage to the superconducting coils, and so a manual quench should only be performed if a person is pinned to the magnet by a large metal object that cannot be removed by hand.

All systems should have helium venting equipment which removes the helium to the outside environment in the event of a quench. However, if this fails, helium vents into the room and replaces oxygen. For this reason, all scan rooms should contain an oxygen monitor that sounds an alarm if the oxygen falls below a certain level.

In case of a quench
- Do not panic.
- Turn on scan room exhaust fan (if not automatically turned on by oxygen monitor).
- Prop open door between operator room and hallway.
- Using the intercom, ask the patient to stay calm and remain on the table. Tell him or her that someone will be in shortly to offer assistance.
- Open window to scan room if so constructed.
- Prop open door to scan room.
- Enter scan room, undock the table, help patient to exit the scan room.
- Evacuate the area until the air is restored to normal.

In case of helium venting

If helium is venting into the room, the scan room door may not open.
- Try opening scan room door several times. If door cannot be opened after 45 seconds, open, or if necessary break, window to scan room to relieve pressure.
- Enter scan room through door. If door does not open, enter through window.
- Evacuate patient as described above.

Magnetic field emergency

If someone is pinned against the magnet by a ferromagnetic object, or if some other magnetic-field related emergency occurs, quench the magnet. A magnet quench will result in several days' downtime, so do not press the button except in a true emergency. Do not attempt to test this button; it should be tested only by qualified service personnel.

Patient emergency

The following groups of patients are at greatest risk for complications during MR scanning:
- Patients likely to develop seizure or claustrophobic reaction.
- Patients with greater than normal potential for cardiac arrest.
- Unconscious, heavily sedated, or confused patients with whom no reliable communication can be maintained.

Since direct observation from the MR operator console is usually partially obscured by the magnet enclosure, be sure to closely monitor these patients at all times to quickly identify and respond to medical emergencies. In some cases, emergency personnel should remain with the patient or be on standby alert to help prevent serious complications or death.

If a patient needs emergency medical attention during the scanning session:
- Hit the Emergency Stop button on the console or magnet enclosure to abort the scan. Notify emergency personnel if necessary. Since ferromagnetic life-support and related equipment cannot be brought into the scan room, it must await the patient outside the scan room.
- Evacuate the patient from the scan room as quickly as possible to a designated emergency medical treatment area outside the exclusion zone.
- Close magnet door.
- Follow hospital emergency protocol.

Safety tips – environment

Here are some tips for maintaining a safe environment for patients and their relatives.

- Before sending the patient an appointment, check with them – or the referring clinician – that they do not have a pacemaker or other contraindicated implants.
- Try to ascertain whether they are likely to suffer from claustrophobia – forewarned is forearmed. But be careful how you question the patient – the mere suggestion of claustrophobia may create the problem itself.
- When sending out the appointment, include any relevant safety information and details of the examination – most of a patient's anxiety is fear of the unknown.
- Try to ensure that the waiting area is calming and pleasant.
- Carefully screen the patient and anyone else accompanying the patient into the scan room. This should include questions about surgical procedures, metal injury to the eye and pacemakers.
- Ensure that the patient and relatives/friends remove all credit cards, loose metal items, keys, jewelry, etc.
- Check for body piercing (any body part can be pierced!).
- Tattoos can heat up during image acquisition. A cool wet cloth placed over the tattoo acts as a good heat dissipater. Tattooed eyeliner may be contraindicated as heat can cause ocular damage.
- Bras and belts should also be removed even if they are non-ferrous and are not in the imaging field. They may still heat up and reduce image quality by locally altering the magnetic field.
- Ask the patient to change into a gown for all examinations, as this is really the only way of ensuring that the patient has removed all dangerous objects.
- Always re-check the patient before they are taken into the magnetic field, regardless of how many times they have been checked before. It is the radiographer's responsibility to keep the MR environment safe.
- Remember that patients may know nothing about magnetism and the potential hazards.
- Anxious and sick patients especially cannot be trusted to give you correct information. Be extra vigilant with these types of patients. If you are in any doubt about their safety DO NOT TAKE THEM INTO THE MAGNETIC FIELD.

Safety tips for dealing with claustrophobic patients

This is a real art and every radiographer, nurse and radiologist has their own way of coaxing a patient into the magnet. Here are a few suggestions:

- Use a mirror so that the patient can see out of the magnet.
- Examine the patient prone when using the body coil.
- Remove the pillow so that the patient's face is further away from the roof of the bore.
- Ask the patient to close their eyes or place a piece of paper towel over their face.
- Tell the patient that they do not have to have the examination and that although MR may be the best way of sorting out their problem, it is by no means the only way. This gives the patient a feeling of control over their own destiny. It is astonishing how many times these few words have worked!
- Bring the patient out of the magnet in between each sequence, especially in long procedures.
- Reassure them that the magnet is open at both ends and that they are not shut in.
- Use the bore light, the air circulation fan and the patient alarm system wherever possible.
- Encourage a relative or friend to accompany them and to maintain physical contact with them throughout the examination.
- Always communicate with the patient during the examination to check that they are OK, and tell them how long the pulse sequences are. Also remember to tell them what is happening in between sequences. There is nothing worse than lying in the magnet and thinking that everyone has gone home and left you.

Appendix 1 Artefacts and their remedies

Artefacts	Axis	Remedy	Penalty
Truncation	phase	respiratory compensation	may lose a slice
		swap phase and frequency	may need anti-aliasing
		gating	variable TR
			variable image contrast
			increased scan time
		pre-saturation	may lose a slice
		gradient moment rephasing	increases minimum TE
Chemical shift	frequency	increase bandwidth	decrease minimum TE available
			decrease SNR
		reduce FOV	reduces SNR
			decreases resolution
		use chemical saturation	reduces SNR
			may lose slices
Chemical misregistration	phase	select a TE at periodicity of fat and water	may lose a slice if TE is significantly reduced
Aliasing	frequency and phase	no frequency wrap	none
		no phase wrap	may reduce SNR
			may increase scan time
			increases motion artefact due to reduced NEX
		enlarge FOV	reduces resolution
Zipper	frequency	call engineer	irate engineer!
Magnetic susceptibility	frequency and phase	use spin echo	not flow sensitive
			blood product may be missed
		remove metal	none
Shading	frequency and phase	check shim	none
		load coil correctly	none
Motion	phase	use antispasmodics	costly
			invasive
		immobilize patient	none
		counseling of patient	none
		all remedies for mismapping	see previous
		sedation	possible side effects
			invasive
			costly
			requires monitoring
Cross talk	slice select	none	none
Cross excitation	slice select	interleaving	doubles the scan time
		squaring off RF pulses	reduces SNR
Moiré	frequency and phase	use SE	none
		patient not to touch bore	none
Magic angle	frequency	change TE	none
		alter position of anatomy	none

Appendix 2 A comparison of acronyms used by manufacturers

	GE	Philips	Siemens	Picker
Spin echo	SE	SE	SE	SE
Fast spin echo	FSE	TSE	TSE	FSE
Inversion recovery	IR	IR	IR	IR
Short Tau inversion recovery	STIR	STIR	STIR	STIR
Fluid attenuated inversion recovery	FLAIR	FLAIR	FLAIR	FLAIR
Coherent gradient echo	GRASS	FFE	FISP	FAST
Incoherent gradient echo	SPGR	T1 FFE	FLASH	RF spoiled FAST
Balanced gradient echo	FIESTA	BFFE	True FISP	–
Steady state free precession	SSFP	T2 FFE	PSIF	CE FAST
Fast gradient echo	Fast GRASS/SPGR	TFE	Turbo FLASH	RAM FAST
Echo planar	EPI	EPI	EPI	EPI
Parallel imaging	ASSET	SENSE	iPAT	SMASH
Spatial pre-saturation	SAT	REST	SAT	Pre-SAT
Gradient moment rephasing	Flow comp	Flow comp	GMR	MAST
Signal averaging	NEX	NSA	AC	NSA
Anti-aliasing	No phase wrap	Foldover suppression	Oversampling	Oversampling
Rectangular FOV	Rect FOV	Rect FOV	Half Fourier imaging	Undersampling
Respiratory compensation	Resp comp	PEAR	Resp trigger	Resp gating

Abbreviations used above

AC	number of acquisitions
ASSET	array spatial and sensitivity encoding technique
CE FAST	contrast enhanced FAST
FAST	Fourier acquired steady state technique
FFE	fast field echo
FIESTA	free induction echo stimulated acquisition
FISP	free induction steady precession
FLAIR	fluid attenuated inversion recovery
FLASH	fast low angled shot
Flow comp	flow compensation
FSE	fast spin echo
GMR	gradient moment rephasing
GRASS	gradient recalled acquisition in the steady state
iPAT	integrated parallel acquisition technique
MAST	motion artefact suppression
MP RAGE	magnetization prepared rapid gradient echo
NEX	number of excitations
NSA	number of signal averages
PEAR	phase encoding artefact reduction
PSIF	mirrored FISP
RAM FAST	rapid acquisition matrix FAST
REST	regional saturation technique
SENSE	sensitivity encoding
SMASH	simultaneous acquisition of spatial harmonics
SPGR	spoiled GRASS
SSFP	steady state free precession
STIR	short tau inversion recovery
TFE	turbo field echo
TSE	turbo spin echo
Turbo FLASH	magnetization prepared sub second imaging

Glossary

2D volumetric acquisition acquisition where a small amount of data is acquired from each slice before repeating the TR

3D volumetric acquisition acquisition where the whole imaging volume is excited so that the images can be viewed in any plane

Actual TE the time between the echo and the next RF pulse in SSFP

Aliasing artefact produced when anatomy outside the FOV is mismapped inside the FOV

Alignment when nuclei are placed in an external magnetic field their magnetic moments line up with the magnetic field flux lines

Alnico alloy that is used to make permanent magnets

Ampere's law determines the magnitude and direction of the magnetic field due to a current; if you point your right thumb along the direction of the current, then the magnetic field points along the direction of the curled fingers

Analogue to digital conversion (ADC) process by which a waveform is sampled and digitized

Angular momentum the spin of MR active nuclei that depends on the balance between the number of protons and neutrons in the nucleus

Anti-parallel alignment describes the alignment of magnetic moments in the opposite direction to the main field

Apparent diffusion coefficient (ADC) net displacement of molecules due to diffusion

Atomic number sum of protons in the nucleus

B$_0$ the main magnetic field measured in tesla

b value strength and duration of diffusion gradients

Balanced gradient echo (BGE) gradient echo sequence that uses balanced gradients and alternating RF pulses

Bipolar describes a magnet with two poles, north and south

Blood oxygen level dependent (BOLD) a functional MRI technique that utilizes the differences in magnetic susceptibility between oxyhaemoglobin and deoxyhaemoglobin to image areas of activated cerebral cortex

Brownian motion internal motion of the molecules

Cardiac gating monitors cardiac electrical activity during the sequence to reduce cardiac wall motion artefact

Central lines area of K space filled with the shallowest phase-encoding slopes

Cerebral blood volume (CBV) volume of blood perfusing through the brain per unit time

Classical theory uses the direction of the magnetic moments to illustrate alignment

Chemical misregistration artefact along the phase axis caused by the phase difference between fat and water

Chemical shift artefact along the frequency axis caused by the frequency difference between fat and water

Co-current flow flow in the same direction as slice excitation

Coherent the magnetic moments of hydrogen are at the same place on the precessional path

Coherent gradient echo (CGE) gradient echo sequence that uses rewinder gradients

Conjugate symmetry symmetry of data in K space

Contrast to Noise ratio (CNR) difference in SNR between two adjacent structures

Countercurrent flow flow in the opposite direction to slice excitation

Cross excitation energy given to nuclei in adjacent slices by the RF pulse

Cross-talk energy given to nuclei in adjacent slices due to spin lattice relaxation

Cryogen bath area around the coils of wire in which cryogens are placed

Cryogens substances used to super cool the coils of wire in a superconducting magnet

Data point digitized data that contains spatial frequency information as a result of spatial encoding

Decay loss of coherent transverse magnetization

Dephasing the magnetic moments of hydrogen are at a different place on their precessional path

Diamagnetism property that shows a small magnetic moment that opposes the applied field

Diffusion a term used to describe moving molecules due to random thermal motion

Diffusion tensor imaging (DTI) DWI sequence that uses very strong multidirectional gradients

Diffusion weighted imaging (DWI) sequence that uses gradients to sensitize the sequence to diffusion

Dixon technique technique that uses a TE when fat and water are out of phase with each other to null the signal from fat

Drive see Fast recovery

Driven equilibrium a sequence that uses an additional pulses to drive any remaining transverse magnetization into the longitudinal plane

Duty cycle the percentage of time a gradient is at maximum amplitude

Echo planar imaging (EPI) sequence that uses single and multishot K space filling techniques with sampling of gradient echoes

Echo spacing spacing between each echo in TSE

Echo train series of 180° rephasing pulse and echoes in a turbo spin echo pulse sequence

Echo train length (ETL) the number of 180° RF pulses and resultant echoes in TSE

Effective TE the time between the echo and the RF pulse that initiated it in SSFP and TSE sequences

Electrons orbit the nucleus in distinct shells and are negatively charged

emf drives a current in a circuit and is the result of a changing magnetic field inducing an electric field

Entry slice phenomena contrast difference of flowing nuclei relative to the stationary nuclei because they are fresh

Excitation the energy transfer from the RF pulse to the NMV

Extrinsic contrast parameters contrast parameters that are controlled by the system operator

Faraday's law of induction law that states that a change of magnetic flux induces an emf in a closed circuit

Fast Fourier transform (FFT) mathematical conversion of frequency/time domain to frequency/amplitude

Fast recovery FSE sequence that uses an additional RF pulse to drive any residual transverse magnetization into the longitudinal plane (also called Drive)

Fast spin echo (FSE) spin echo sequence that decreases scan time by filling multiple lines of K space every TR (also called turbo spin echo)

Ferromagnetism property of a substance that ensures that it remains magnetic, is permanently magnetized and subsequently becomes a permanent magnet

Field of view (FOV) area of anatomy covered in an image

FLAIR (fluid attenuated inversion recovery) IR sequences that nulls the signal from CSF

Fleming's right-hand rule see Ampere's law

Flip angle the angle of the NMV to B_0

Flow compensation see Gradient moment nulling

Flow encoding axes axes along which bipolar gradients act in order to sensitize flow along the axis of the gradient; used in phase contrast MRA

Flow phenomena artefacts produced by flowing nuclei

Flow-related enhancement decrease in time of flight due to a decrease in velocity of flow

Free induction decay (FID) loss of signal due to relaxation

Frequency the speed with which a spin precesses or a waveform oscillates

Frequency encoding locating a signal according to its frequency

Frequency matrix number of pixels in the frequency direction of an image

Frequency shift difference in frequency between spins located along a gradient

Fresh spins nuclei that have not been beaten down by repeated RF pulses

Fringe field stray magnetic field outside the bore of the magnet

Functional MR imaging (fMRI) a rapid MR imaging technique that acquires images of the brain during activity or stimulus and at rest

Gadolinium (Gd) positive contrast agent

Gauss (G) unit of field strength; 1 tesla = 10,000 gauss

Ghosting motion artefact in the phase axis

Gradient amplifier supplies power to the gradient coils

Gradient echo pulse sequence one that uses a gradient to regenerate an echo

Gradient echo (GE) echo produced as a result of gradient rephasing

Gradient moment nulling (GMN) uses additional gradients to reduce flow artefact

Gradient spoiling the use of gradients to dephase magnetic moments; the opposite of rewinding

Gradients coils of wire that alter the magnetic field strength in a linear fashion when a current is passed through them

Gyromagnetic ratio the precessional frequency of an element at 1.0 T

High velocity signal loss increase in time of flight due to an increase in the velocity of flow

Homogeneity the evenness of the magnetic field

Hybrid sequences sequences where a series of gradient echoes are interspersed 180° rephasing pulses; in this way susceptibility artefacts are reduced

Hyperintense high signal intensity (bright)

Hypointense low signal intensity (dark)

Incoherent means that the magnetic moments of hydrogen are at different places on the precessional path

Incoherent gradient echo gradient echo sequence that uses RF spoiling for T1 weighting

Induced electric current oscillating current that occurs when a magnet is moved in a closed circuit

Inflow effect another term for entry slice phenomenon

Inhomogeneities areas where the magnetic field strength is not exactly the same as the main field strength

Intravoxel dephasing phase difference between flow and stationary nuclei in a voxel

Intrinsic contrast mechanisms contrast parameters that do not come under the operator's control

Inversion recovery (IR) sequence that uses an inverting pulse to saturate or null tissue

Ions atoms with an excess or deficit of electrons

Isointense same signal intensity

Isotopes atoms of the same element having a different mass number

J coupling a process that describes the reduction the spin-spin interactions in fat, thereby increasing its T2 decay time

Kilogauss (kG) unit of field strength (1000 gauss)

K space an area where raw data is stored

Larmor equation used to calculate the frequency or speed of precession for a specific nucleus in a specific magnetic field strength

Lenz's law states that induced emf is in a direction so that it opposes the change in magnetic field which causes it

Longitudinal plane the axis parallel to B_0

Magnetic flux density number of flux lines per unit area

Magnetic isocentre the centre of the bore of the magnet in all planes

Magnetic lines of flux lines of force running from the magnetic south to the north poles of the magnet

Magnetic moment denotes the direction of the north/south axis of a magnet and the amplitude of the magnetic field

Magnetic susceptibility ability of a substance to become magnetized

Magnetism a property of all matter that depends on the magnetic susceptibility of the atom

Magnetization prepared a prepulse applied before the main sequence to null the signal from certain tissues in fast gradient echo

Magnetization transfer transfer of RF energy from free to bound protons

Magnitude image unsubtracted image combination of flow sensitized data

Mass number sum of neutrons and protons in the nucleus

Mean transit time (MTT) used in perfusion imaging to indicate the transit time of blood through a tissue

MR active nuclei that possess an odd number of protons

MR angiography method of visualizing vessels that contain flowing nuclei by producing a contrast between them and the stationary nuclei

MR signal the voltage induced in the receiver coil

Multishot (MS) technique that fills K space in multiple sections

Net magnetization vector (NMV) the magnetic vector produced as a result of the alignment of excess hydrogen nuclei with B_0

Neutrons particles in the nucleus that have no charge

Null point point at which there is no longitudinal magnetization in a tissue

Number of signal averages (NSA) the number of times an echo is encoded with the same slope of phase-encoding gradient

Nyquist theorem states that frequencies must be sampled at a rate at least twice that of the highest frequency in the echo in order to reliably reproduce it

Off resonant RF pulses applied at a frequency slightly different to the Larmor frequency of a tissue

On resonant RF pulses applied at the Larmor frequency of a particular tissue

Outer lines area of K space filled with the steepest phase-encoding gradient slopes

Out-of-phase artefact see Chemical misregistration

Parallel alignment describes the alignment of magnetic moments in the same direction as the main field

Parallel imaging technique that uses multiple coils to fill multiple lines of K space every TR

Paramagnetism property whereby substances affect external magnetic fields in a positive way, resulting in a local increase in the magnetic field

Partial averaging filling only a proportion of K space with data and putting zeroes in the remainder

Partial echo sampling only part of the echo and extrapolating the remainder in K space

Perfusion a measure of the quality of vascular supply to a tissue

Permanent magnets magnets which retain their magnetism

Phase the position of a magnetic moment on its precessional path at any given time

Phase contrast angiography technique that generates vascular contrast by applying a bipolar gradient to different stationary and moving spins by their phase

Phase encoding locating a signal according to its phase

Phase image subtracted image combination of flow sensitized data

Phase matrix number of pixels in the phase direction of an image

Phase shift difference in phase between spins located along a gradient

Pixel picture element in the FOV

Polarity the direction of a gradient i.e. which end is greater than B_0 and which is lower than B_0; depends on the direction of the current through the gradient coil

Precession the secondary spin of magnetic moments around B_0

Precessional frequency frequency with which MR active nuclei precess when exposed to an external magnetic field

Presaturation technique that uses RF pulses before the sequence to null the signal from moving spins or from certain types of tissue

Protium isotope of hydrogen that has a mass and atomic number of 1; MR active nucleus used in MRI

Protons particles in n the nucleus that are positively charged

Proton density the number of protons in a unit volume of tissue

Proton density weighting image that demonstrates the differences in the proton densities of the tissues

Pulse control unit coordinates the switching on and off of the gradient and RF transmitter coils at appropriate times during the pulse sequence

Pulse sequence a series of RF pulses, gradients applications and intervening time periods; used to control contrast

Quantum theory uses the energy level of the nuclei to illustrate alignment

Quenching process by which there is a sudden loss of the superconductivity of the magnet coils so that the magnet becomes resistive

Radiowaves waves of electromagnetic radiation that have a oscillate with a radiofrequency

Ramp sampling where sampling data points are collected when the gradient rise time is almost complete; sampling occurs while the gradient is still reaching maximum amplitude, while the gradient is at maximum amplitude, and as it begins to decline

Readout gradient the frequency-encoding gradient

Receive bandwidth range of frequencies that are sampled during readout; determines the sampling rate

Recovery growth of longitudinal magnetization

Rectangular FOV FOV where the phase FOV is smaller than the frequency FOV

Relaxation process by which the NMV loses energy

Relaxivity process by which relaxation rates of a tissue are altered by administering contrast agents

Repetition time (TR) time between each excitation pulse

Rephasing creating in phase magnetization, usually by using an RF pulse or a gradient

Residual magnetization transverse magnetization left over from previous RF pulses in steady state conditions

Resistive magnet an electromagnet created by passing current through loops of wire

Resonance an energy transition that occurs when an object is subjected to a frequency the same as its own

Respiratory compensation uses bellows around the patient's chest to reduce respiratory motion artefact

Rewinding the use of a gradient to rephase magnetic moments

RF amplifier supplies power to the RF transmitter coils

RF pulse short burst of RF energy which excites nuclei into a high energy state

RF spoiling the use of digitized RF to transmit and receive at a certain phase

RF transmitter coil coil that transmits RF at the resonant frequency of hydrogen to excite nuclei and move them into a high energy state

Rise time the time it takes a gradient to switch on, achieve the required gradient slope, and switch off again

Sampling rate rate at which samples are taken during readout

Sampling time the time that the readout gradient is switched on for

Saturation occurs when the NMV is flipped to a full $180°$

Sequential acquisition acquisition where all the data from each slice is acquired before going onto the next

Shim coil extra coils used to make the magnetic filed as homogeneous as possible

Shimming process whereby the evenness of the magnetic field is optimized

Signal to noise ratio (SNR) ratio of signal relative to noise

Single shot (SS) a sequence where all the lines of K space are acquire at once

Slew rate function of gradient rise time and amplitude

Slice encoding the separation of individual slice locations by phase in volume acquisitions

Slice selection selecting a slice using a gradient

Spatial encoding spatially locating a signal in three dimensions

Spatial resolution the ability to distinguish two points as separate

Specific absorption rate (SAR) rate/kg at which energy from the RF pulse is dissipated

Spectroscopy provides a frequency spectrum of a given tissue based on the molecular and chemical structures of that tissue

Spin down the population of high-energy hydrogen nuclei that align their magnetic moments antiparallel to the main field

Spin echo pulse sequence one that uses a $180°$ rephasing pulse to generate an echo

Spin echo (SE) echo produced as a result of a $180°$ rephasing pulse

Spin lattice relaxation process by which energy is given up to the surrounding lattice

Spin-spin relaxation process by which interactions between the magnetic fields of adjacent nuclei cause dephasing

Spin up the population of low energy hydrogen nuclei that align their magnetic moments parallel to B_0

Spoiling a process of dephasing spins either with a gradient or an RF pulse

Steady State a situation when the TR is shorter than both the T1 and T2 relaxation times of all the tissues

Steady state free precession (SSFP) gradient echo sequence that uses echo shifting for T2 weighting

Stimulated echo echo produced by previous RF pulse in a steady state sequence by rephasing residual transverse magnetization

Stimulated-echo acquisition mode (STEAM) technique used in spectroscopy

STIR (short TI inversion recovery) sequence used to suppress fat

Superconducting magnet electromagnet that use supercooled coils of wire so that there is no inherent resistance in the system; the current flows, and therefore the magnetism is generated without a driving voltage

T1 recovery growth of longitudinal magnetization as a result of spin lattice relaxation

T1 recovery time time taken for 63% of the longitudinal magnetization to recover

T1 weighted image image that demonstrates the differences in the T1 times of the tissues

T2 decay loss of coherent transverse magnetization as a result of spin-spin relaxation

T2 decay time time taken for 63% of the transverse magnetization to decay

T2 weighted image image that demonstrates the differences in the T2 times of the tissues

T2* dephasing due to inhomogeneities

Time from Inversion (TI) time between inversion and excitation in IR sequences

Tesla (T) unit of field strength

Time intensity curve used in perfusion imaging to measure perfusion kinetics of a volume of tissue

Time-of-flight angiography (TOF MRA) technique that generates vascular contrast by utilizing the inflow effect

Time of flight rate of flow in a given time; causes some flowing nuclei to receive one RF pulse only and therefore produce a signal void

Time to echo (TE) time between the excitation pulse and the echo

Transceiver coil that both transmits RF and receives the MR signal

Transmit bandwidth range of frequencies transmitted in an RF pulse

Transverse plane the axis perpendicular to B_0

Turbo factor or echo train length the number of 180° rephasing pulse/echoes/phase encodings per TR in fast spin echo

Turbo spin echo (TSE) see Fast spin echo

Velocity encoding (VENC) sensitizes the sequence to blood flow in PC MRA

Volume coil coil that transmits and receives signal over a large volume of the patient

Voxel volume of tissue in the patient

Voxel volume size of a voxel

Watergram TSE sequence using very long TRs, TEs and turbo factors to produce very heavy T2 weighting

Weighting process by which parameters are manipulated so that one intrinsic contrast mechanism is more dominant than the others

Index